HIDDEN SECRE[T]
CHRONIC DISEASE

Natalia

No one will try
harder to get you better
than the West clinic.

Thanks for coming

Dr West

HIDDEN SECRETS TO CURING YOUR
CHRONIC DISEASE

Real Science,
Real Solution,
and Real Stories
of Healing and Hope

DR. JASON WEST
DC NMD FIAMA DCDBN

He who has his health has a thousand dreams; he who does not has only one.

~ Arabian proverb

Table of Contents

1

HOW TO GET THE MOST
OUT OF THIS BOOK

FOR THE CHRONICALLY sick patient, this book is going to change your life. There are many health books today, but this one is different because until now much of what is in this book wasn't possible for you to access. The treatments I am going to tell you about were developed through 100 years of treating patients. My great-grandfather taught my grandfather, grandfather taught dad, and dad taught me. There isn't another clinic like ours in the USA and probably not in the world.

These are the HIDDEN SECRETS to curing your chronic disease.

You are going to get a big dose of vitamin H (Hope). This isn't a real vitamin but the experiences of other people are intended to give you the most important vitamin...Hope. I love this saying;

He who has health has hope, and he who has hope has everything.

~ Arabian proverb.

I am so passionate about this that I publish a blog about it— www.dailydosevitaminh.com

I know you are super busy, overwhelmed and looking for ways to get healthy. My guess is that you have seen a lot of doctors, got a lot of opinions, and have tried a whole bunch of things to get healthy but if it would have worked for you or your loved one, you wouldn't be reading this book.

THE MOST IMPORTANT ASSET WE HAVE IS HEALTH. The most important asset we have is health. Just ask anyone that is struggling with their health or just as important, talk to a husband or wife whose spouse is ill. I see this all the time in successful, type A personalities that are enormously successful monetarily but have sacrificed their health for financial or business success. In the end these people trade some or all of their money for their health.

If you are healthy you can always work to regain and maintain relationships, to rebuild your life, and fill your bank account. If you have chronic disease, willpower can only take you so far. This leads me to the next important discussion.

There is a lot of terrible information about health. Diseases, especially in the chronic disease category, are not treated effectively with prescriptive medications and surgery, and yet, that is what most people are taught. Also there is doctor Google, this amazing and detrimental information source. Amazing because of the information available and detrimental because of the misinformation available.

While you are reading this book, I encourage you to keep an open mind. There is a century of in the trenches information from successfully treating patients. This is so important because when you help Mrs.

Smith with a treatment protocol, and then do it on hundreds of patients across decades of time, you know that the protocol helps people.

Please remember this—just because you haven't heard of the treatment, doesn't mean that it doesn't work, it just means you haven't heard of it. Don't let your education get in the way of your intelligence. We all look at the world through a layer of experience, education and bias. So many times people are taught to think or view something that is not accurate.

I have seen firsthand the protocols, treatments and therapies in this book help improve nearly everyone, not necessarily cure, but nearly always improve quality of life. Sometimes people have waited for so long or sometimes their body is too far ravaged with disease to help them. However, I have seen these patient's quality of life improve. I love providing this type of health care.

<u>Step 1</u> - Take responsibility for your health. In some instances this is easier said than done. It may not be your fault, you may be the victim of an accident, some bad DNA, bad genes or just bad luck. Sometimes a genetic disease may not be improved, but the decision of how you live your life is only made by you.

<u>Step 2</u> - Learn all you can about your body, symptoms, conditions, treatments and available options. In the financial world there's a saying: no one likes your money as much as you. It's the same about your health, no one likes your health as much as you.

<u>Step 3</u> - Access the source of vitamin H (vitamin hope). The first thing you should do is to sign up for the free videos, reports and information on the website: www.hiddensecretscure.com

One of the benefits you will receive when you register is free video updates and book notification updates (remember, I am relentless in finding new treatments, protocols and breakthroughs.) Having a cutting-edge clinic is a work in progress and we are always searching for the best treatments for our patients.

Register for updates on our patient blog www.dailydosevitaminh. com. Nothing provides more hope to you or your loved one than to hear success stories from other patients from all over the world. We have hundreds of satisfied patient outcomes.

<u>Step 4</u> - Attend one of our educational events on the Internet. These high-quality events cover topics like:

- Lyme disease
- Fibromyalgia
- Macular degeneration
- Peripheral neuropathy
- The arthritis cure
- Asthma
- Diabetes
- Stomach problems of all types

If you are signed up for information on the book website or the patient blog you will automatically get notified of these events.

<u>Step 5</u> - I am a big believer in patient intuition. I believe patients know their bodies better than doctors. Learn all you can about your condition. It doesn't matter who gets the credit or what treatment you do as long as you get better. Read whatever jumps out and speaks to you, trust your intuition and your gut as I do. Many times the best patient outcomes I have achieved are because I listened to that intuition.

Nothing is more empowering than to achieve and maintain optimal health. Think of this as an investment, read, study, and ask about your health.

The #1 lesson to walk away with from this book is when you balance your physiology, your emotions, your hormones, your energy, and your bio mechanics—you now have a chance to live the healthy life you desire. It's all about balance.

I am going to share transformational patient stories that will help you learn more about your condition and give you hope that you can be healthy. You'll be inspired by the patient stories and use the stories and treatments in your own health pursuits.

The protocols in this book work—I have seen it my whole life. I grew up in the Clinic and have spent my whole professional career learning the best treatments for chronic diseases.

THE PROTOCOLS IN THIS BOOK WORK...

A Warning

There's never a good time to be sick. It's so frustrating to outline a treatment program for a patient and they don't take action. Frequently they return months or years later with the same illness. Had they followed the program, they would have been on the path to recovery. It's also more affordable than waiting for the perfect set of circumstances.

A Promise

I routinely see miracles, matter of fact; we jokingly said we were going to rename the West Clinic, the Clinic of Spontaneous Remission. This was after I saw a note from a doctor that had been managing a chronic disease and the patient came to our clinic and got better. The patient made great progress and her doctor wrote, "Observing the patient for non-prescriptive spontaneous remission." Another patient told me his doctor told him this, "There's no way that stuff Dr. West is doing does anything, but a lot of people go there and seem to get better. It's really just placebo." The patient told me, "I told the doctor that perhaps he should get some of the placebo medicine."

If you follow the recommendations in this book by taking accountability, educating yourself on your options and balancing your body's biochemistry, biomechanics, hormones, energy, and emotions, then improved health is in your future.

Let's not focus on the past treatment failures; instead let's work on life from here forward. With your health, you can accomplish all of your dreams. Let's get started.

2

A STORY OF HOPE –
AMANDA

HOW I LOST and then regained my hope, my health and my life. It was 5:30 am and I was in the middle of endless seizures and struggling to breathe. I remember the feeling that I wouldn't make it through the night and was doing everything I could to stay awake, to avoid never waking up again. I was lying on the couch. My mom was across from me because I couldn't be left alone. I picked up my iPad and did the best I could to write goodbye letters to everyone I loved because I didn't think I'd have a chance to speak to them again...

Three years before that, I never thought a tick bite would almost end my life. I was a perfectly healthy 15-year-old girl. I stayed active, played soccer, loved reading and going to school. I'd never imagined that one morning on May 11, 2012 when I woke up in bed with the flu that it would take three years and hundreds of thousands of dollars to recover.

I'm now 19 years old and even though I've had Lyme disease for more than 14 years, I was only diagnosed in July of 2012 after begging the doctor to sign off an order indicating I had Lyme. When I was five years old, my family was camping out in the Ocala National Forest in Florida. During that time, I got bit by a tick and within weeks I started having symptoms that would drag on for the next six years. I started having an autoimmune reaction called vitiligo where my skin turned white on many different spots on my body. I had extreme vision loss, headaches, stomach aches, fainting spells, and extreme joint pain to the point that I couldn't walk for weeks at a time. I blacked out at school, had memory loss, forgetfulness, numbness, shooting pain throughout my body, and fatigue. The TMJ in my jaw got so bad that I was unable to open my mouth for more than 10 months.

When I was about 12 years old, my symptoms started to subside and for about a year and a half I was almost symptom free. Of course I had a headache here and there, my vision didn't get better, but it was no longer getting worse, and my joints would ache from time to time, but it was the best I'd felt in years.

In the summer of 2010, I was 14 years old. I started working on our family farm almost every day, feeding the animals, picking things in the field. I was outside almost all day, every day in the tall grass. There were ticks all the time, but we thought nothing of it. When school started back up, I went from a straight A student, reading more than 50 books during the summer and not having to work very hard, to having a very hard time doing anything. My mom noticed that I was having trouble concentrating. Things were much harder for me to do. I was ditzy and not understanding things or getting jokes as quickly as I did before. I started getting sick again.

* * *

I had strep throat three times over the course of five months. I was playing soccer for my school and I noticed that I was having a lot more trouble keeping up with the other girls doing the exercises. I was getting much more worn out than I had been in years before. When soccer ended, I started doing P90X and stuck with it. I was having symptoms that I should've noticed, but I just placed it in the back of my mind as I did not want to get sick again. But then I woke up one morning and told my mom I just didn't feel right. I couldn't handle noise or light. I had headaches, joint pain, vision problems, and chest pain. I was confused and couldn't keep up with conversations. I slept 18 hours a day.

All of my symptoms were back, but much worse than before. My mom was alarmed at the way I looked. Just overnight I looked so sick and frail. She took me to my doctor. They ran some tests but there was nothing wrong. My symptoms got worse. I was no longer able to get out of bed. I couldn't walk upstairs, I was unable to eat and I lost 30 pounds. My symptoms were scary, **NOBODY HAD ANY IDEA WHAT WAS WRONG WITH ME. I HONESTLY THOUGHT I WOULD DIE.** to say the least. Nobody had any idea what was wrong with me. I honestly thought I would die. I'd seen over 60 doctors since I was six and none of them had been able to tell me what was wrong. It got to a point where I went to my mom and requested to have all of my medical records sent to our house so that I could look through them. Within two weeks of being able to look over every bit of my records, I made charts, circling and highlighting information. I came to the conclusion that I had Lyme disease. My parents and I watched a documentary on Lyme disease entitled "Under Our Skin". This confirmed my conclusion.

Two weeks later, after begging a doctor to sign off on an order, I had a positive test result for Lyme disease. I was so relieved and happy to finally have an answer, but I had no idea the troubles I would face getting treatment. I was looking forward to being healthy again.

I had two positive tests and all the symptoms of Lyme's, even a bull's-eye rash. Doctors still refused to believe that I had Lyme disease. I got to the point that I was no longer able to walk or read. I had days that I couldn't even speak or handle any kind of light or noise, and had hundreds of seizures. The Lyme had spread to my brain, my heart, my muscles, my bones, my organs...to every part of my body. The oxygen and blood flow to my brain had slowed. A SPECT scan even confirmed that it was from the Lyme disease. Doctors told me it was all in my head, that I was crazy and depressed. They told me I needed to see a psychiatrist. They said anything as long as they did not have to admit that I had Lyme disease and didn't have to treat me. Doctors shouldn't be scared to treat somebody with a very real condition because they fear they'll get their license taken away. This is affecting many more people than we know. It's ruining lives. Doctors have tried telling me that I have multiple sclerosis, chronic fatigue, fibromyalgia, Lupus, and arthritis, without ever having a positive test result. But I had two positive test results for Lyme disease and they told me I didn't have it.

Three years into this illness, I'd reached my lowest point. I'd lost all of my friends. I was alone. I was sick. I'd gotten to the point that I couldn't feed myself, bathe myself, or get dressed. At times I was unable to talk and couldn't even recognize my own family. Every day was a fight to survive, a fight that was slowly draining me. Every breath was a struggle and doctors suggested putting me on a feeding tube and leaving me in the hospital because I wouldn't get better. I honestly never thought I would. I had prepared myself to die, as hard as it was and as much as I wanted to live. Fighting was too hard and I was ready to be put out of my misery. However, one day my uncle was listening to "Seasons on the Fly." Greg Heister was talking about the West Clinic and the treatment he was receiving for Lyme disease.

After my uncle told my parents about the clinic, they immediately started researching it. My parents made the decision that my mom and I would move to Idaho, splitting up our family for six months in a last ditch effort to save my life. We didn't have any options left and even though we'd spent so much money already, we finally saw a glimpse of hope. I never expected to get better or to walk again. I was extremely skeptical, but after getting to the clinic, meeting Dr. J, and getting treatment every day, I slowly started feeling better and better. It was hard to believe since I'd seen improvement with other treatments, only to plateau or get sick again. But at the West Clinic, I just kept getting better and healthier. Soon I began reading and writing again. My seizures stopped, and at the end of five months, I took my first steps in two years. Two years!

It's been a year since I started walking and getting back to living a normal life. I got my GED after missing so much high school and am going on to hopefully become a physician's assistant and help others the way Dr. J helped me.

Missy Tomazin - Our Journey Near Hopelessness

I've been a Christian for 20 years. I met my husband shortly after salvation and we knew right away that we wanted to get married and start a family. Paul and I had four children in just under five years; twin girls and then two boys. Our oldest daughter, Amanda, has experienced oddities in her health since she was 5 years old. Through the years, some issues seemed far more serious and others were more of a nuisance than anything else; nothing life-threatening. For instance, in first grade she developed vitiligo. She would pass out in the heat and dislocate joints easily. She had unexplainable cold extremities, constant headaches, and drastic changes in vision. For over a year she often battled strep throat, Mononucleosis, random fevers, lockjaw and didn't sweat. It was sort of a roller coaster ride of not knowing what was coming or when. We saw a plethora of doctors through those early years and many times we were told that she would likely outgrow the symptoms. They were never able to tell us why she seemed to be having so many problems. They also didn't think any of these were at all related. They were simply coincidental.

Then she sailed through a few good years without anything significant. She played soccer for a couple of years, but would experience moments of extreme fatigue. Her lifestyle became far more active and she was determined; things seemed to be going really well for her. She was engaged in an intense workout program called P90X, that conditioned her for the upcoming soccer season. She was busy helping around the family vegetable farm and excelling in school. We thought the worst was behind her. Well, we certainly hoped the worst was behind her. We were wrong. She was 15 years old and nearly finished with her freshman year of high school when one Friday morning she woke up not feeling well; everything hurt. We didn't think too much of it and she spent the weekend in bed. Over the next few days, her symptoms worsened. We took her to the doctor, suspecting the flu. We were told it was a virus that needed to run its course.

DAYS TURNED INTO WEEKS AND WEEKS TURNED INTO MONTHS

Days turned into weeks and weeks turned into months and this "virus" wasn't going away on its' own. After a couple of months, Amanda's lack of strength and energy to do anything other than sleep did not improve. We began pursuing answers. In those first couple of months we had many doctors' appointments, procedures, ER visits, and prescriptions for various ailments. Each time we hoped for answers, help, direction and encouragement. Every single time ended with disappointment and feelings of defeat. Tests were inconclusive, doctors were accusatory of us as parents and often berated us and Amanda. At best, prescriptions seemed to worsen the symptoms. We often received direction to pursue another specialist and were almost always told to seek a psychologist because it was likely all in her head! We started doubting everything and felt like we were going crazy. We began to realize that if we wanted answers, we would need to take matters into our own hands and venture outside of traditional medical practices.

There has been a multitude of possible diseases or disorders that Amanda was tested for. Everything was inconclusive. After some discussions with friends, we began researching Lyme disease and thought maybe that was what Amanda had. We sat down as a family and watched "Under Our Skin." For the first time since that dreadful day in May, so much seemed to make sense. After more research, we sent a sample of Amanda's blood away to be tested by a reputable lab on the west coast. By the end of July, we received a positive test result for Lyme disease. We were rejoicing over finally having an answer. That rejoicing was short lived though. We quickly came to realize that simply having a diagnosis for Lyme by no means insured proper treatment. We began to see that the very term was extremely controversial and seemed taboo among medical doctors. After more education on Lyme and treatment options, we opted to pursue an aggressive antibiotic protocol that entailed traveling to see a specialist in New York. We were committed to the treatment. However, long distance care from a specialist in New York, while living in Florida wasn't effective for us. There was no doctor in Florida willing to watch over Amanda while she was receiving this treatment. Our local doctors wanted no part of it. She quickly showed signs of improvement, then rapidly declined. Her body seemed to be shutting down. We managed to get some labs on her and they were awful. We stopped all antibiotics immediately. We were doing the detox methods, but it was nowhere close to what was needed. Amanda was on a slippery slope. She was frail!

Let me try to paint a picture for you... She had lost all muscle tone. Her appetite was gone, she weighed 88 pounds. The smell of food made her nauseous. She had constant stomach pains. She never sat at the table with us to share a meal anymore. Her headache was constant and varied in intensity. She had no energy, or was in bed, 95% of the time. She was hyper-sensitive to lights and sounds. Inside our home with shades and curtains pulled, she wore dark prescription sunglasses. Most often a lamp was overwhelming. She couldn't tolerate noise or even voices. A whisper was often too much, not to mention the sound of whistling or music (or life happening in a family of six). When she would watch TV with the family, it was with closed captioning on. She could no longer read (which was a love of hers). She could no longer write, form letters or even spell words, written or verbal. Her comprehension had plummeted. She was unable to make sense of simple statements and no longer knew the meaning or context of basic words. Seeking to communicate about anything brought great frustration and discouragement. Her joints ached all the time. She had odd zaps of aches and pains that flooded her body. Still, no assistance was available from local medical doctors.

* * *

We were consumed with medical expenses. Anything that seemed to help in any way, shape or form didn't seem to be covered by insurance. Our amazing family, friends and community rallied around us to plan a fundraiser. Just one week before the event, my brother-in-law happened to hear a snippet about the West Clinic and Lyme disease on ESPNs "Seasons on the Fly", by host Greg Heister. My brother-in-law told us about it the same day.

We visited the website, listened to some testimonials and called the office. Alicia, Dr. Jason West's assistant, got my message of sheer desperation and called me back that evening. She listened to me, answered all my questions, comforted me, and assured me we were not alone, nor were we crazy. She was able to work us in as an emergency case and we were in their office just a few days later, in Idaho!

Amanda, Haley (Amanda's twin sister) and I missed the fundraiser because we were on a plane bound for Idaho that very day. The money coming in made it possible, due to the incredible financial support and sacrifice from so many loving people. We spent three weeks there. I was so encouraged!

Amanda felt too bad to feel any sense of encouragement. Traveling had been very difficult on her. We met Dr. Jason West and he answered all our questions and listened to us...really listened to us. We fully believed that God had led us to Idaho to heal Amanda. While at the West Clinic, Amanda received treatment we'd never heard of before. Some of the treatments she responded to really well, some she didn't simply because she was so weak and frail. Dr. J tailored her treatment to meet her needs. There wasn't a standard protocol that was meant for everyone. I was extremely encouraged and optimistic. We saw Amanda moving in a positive direction for the first time since May. We returned home two days before Christmas with a protocol to continue at home and plans to return to the West Clinic.

As 2013 began, things seemed to be looking up. We had all the supplies we needed and there was a good line of communication with the Clinic. Just a few months into home treatment, we found ourselves in the midst of another one of life's trials. We were now facing another life-threatening issue with another one of our children. So as life goes, everything else was put on hold until she was out of the woods and no longer in danger. That seemed to take longer than anticipated but thankfully, she was doing significantly better and we were grateful.

* * *

Once back on track, we had more blood work done on Amanda and began to realize that she wasn't doing as well back home as she had been doing in Idaho. Idaho was across the country. We wrestled with how we could facilitate her getting the necessary treatment, and it seemed impossible to us. I was needed at home in Florida, my kids needed me, my husband needed me, we didn't have the money...we didn't know what to do. So we continued to research options, and we researched and researched. Little by little by little Amanda continued to decline. We had begun another bout with doctors and hospitals and facilities to no avail. Amanda had now lost the ability to stand up. She could no longer walk at all, not even take a single step, not even with assistance. She was in a wheelchair. She was experiencing seizure-like activity all day long, but it was far more severe at night. She experienced short-term memory loss. At times she did not recognize her siblings or even us, her parents. This was especially terrifying to her but to us as well. Every night she'd lose her ability to talk and would have to communicate through sign language and hand gestures. Her blood pressure was too low for comfort. She had insomnia every night from 8:00 p.m.-4:00 am. She began experiencing difficulty breathing. To assist Amanda, we installed a handicap bar in our living room. She used the frame of her bed to hang on to, giving her a sense of comfort in taking breaths. Her bladder and kidneys would not allow her to properly void. She had a constant urge to urinate and wasn't able to full empty her bladder. Her voice was weak. She kept an iPad or iPhone with her at all times to aid in communication. She often described her heart as cramping. She could not be left alone and required someone with her around the clock. She no longer had any friends coming to visit, which ultimately seemed best because she couldn't tolerate visits anyway. She was isolated and we had also become isolated.

We really found ourselves completely overwhelmed. We arrived at a point of just being able to function. It became difficult to think and process where we were, how we came to this point, and thought *what in the world could we do now*. Today, I'm unsure how the ball began rolling again, I just know that it did.

WHAT IN THE WORLD COULD WE DO NOW?

In the spring of 2015, my husband and I knew that without divine intervention, we would be planning a funeral within a year. With the support of a dear friend, we began raising money once again. Our church family was a huge support financially and spiritually, and had been all along. At this point, drastic measures were necessary. We believed that if Amanda had any hope of a future here on this earth, we would need to separate our family. Amanda and I would need to move to Idaho for awhile. This was not an easy decision to make, however we felt it was our only option. We began making plans and once again the Lord provided. In July 2015, we were back in Idaho to pursue treatment at the West Clinic. This time, for a much longer period. I think everyone but Amanda was optimistic. At this point, she was angry and ready to die. Part of her wanted to. She felt death taking over her body...nothing brought her joy anymore. She simply existed. Prior to moving to Idaho, she had written goodbye letters to each of us; me, her dad and her siblings. She didn't think she would win this battle.

We arrived in Idaho and began treatment all over again. It was exciting to see Dr. J and Alicia and the rest of the staff again, but it was also very humbling. I felt like a terrible mom. I wrestled with lots of "if only" thoughts. I could answer all the questions that plagued my mind as to why it had taken so long to get back to Idaho, but that no longer mattered. It was time to put that behind me and press on. We were there for the long haul. We were back to that very point in December 2012, where we saw just a glimpse of improvement. Dr. J is dedicated to continuing education. He is constantly learning. This time, as we sat before him, he told us that he was much better at what he does now because of what he's learned. He also had another doctor in the office and they worked beautifully together. I really felt that we were exactly where we needed to be. We were in good hands. That Tuesday in the office confirmed to me that Amanda really was as bad as I thought she was, if not worse. So we spent time with Dr. J and Dr. Vance and came up with a plan of action. We were in the office every day and spent from 4 to 9 hours there, every time. The days were long and exhausting, but that's what we were there for. My experience in the IV room was priceless. I met amazing people that were sick and would openly discuss

DR. J IS DEDICATED TO CONTINUING EDUCATION. HE IS CONSTANTLY LEARNING.

what was wrong with them, how they felt, what treatment they were receiving, what they've tried, where they were from, where they'd been for treatment, the impact of sickness on their family, supplemental devices and machines they'd purchased for home use. They told of tests and lab work that had been helpful, techniques they did at home, how they seemed to be responding to treatment, what worked for them and what didn't, how long they'd been sick, their hopes and dreams...even their fears. To read this may sound depressing, but more often than not I walked away encouraged. Many times our hearts were knitted together and friendships were formed. There were many times that I had nothing to say to the heartbroken person sitting near me, and all I could do was pray for them.

Quite frequently when someone is extremely ill, others can see improvement before the sick person ever feels it, or is willing to acknowledge it. Looking back at my notes, we were there exactly one month when I started seeing improvement. Paul had flown out for a surprise visit. He was able to see the same improvements I had seen. Amanda was more willing to engage in conversations with others. Before now she would sit in a recliner at the clinic with her dark sunglasses and ear plugs or headphones and zone out. She felt terrible and was too overly stimulated to simply sit in the same room with everyone else. Her bladder and kidneys seemed to be functioning better, her breathing had improved and she was smiling a little easier.

However, when we would comment on how she seemed to be doing a little better or even looked better, she would become very annoyed. What we didn't quite understand then was that she had been hopeful so many times about getting better, only to lose hope when she got worse. She was sure that would happen again, and she would not let herself get excited about feeling better, even when she saw improvement.

Dr. Hollingsworth, another amazing piece of the puzzle and part of the dynamic team at the West Clinic, met with Amanda at least twice a month, sometimes more. Her time spent with him was worth its' weight in gold. He was seeking to help Amanda's body and mind embrace the idea of returning to good health and functioning as God designed our bodies to function. He broke through layer after layer. He too, was a blessing.

Due to some test results we got back, Amanda began a new prescription, some new supplements and began getting methylcobalamin shots. With this new protocol in addition to the IV bags Dr. J was having mixed for Amanda, we saw an almost immediate change. She was different. She was getting her strength back. She had done whatever floor exercises she could all along, during her hours of insomnia, although now they had become more intense and she did them daily. She started having an appetite. She had always loved to cook and began doing that again. She was willing to go to dinner or shopping... we even went to the movies!!! This was huge! Amanda was willing to admit for the first time that she was getting better. Her sister flew out to Idaho to spend some time with her. That allowed me the opportunity to fly home to see the rest of the family and have a little break from our routine. This was needful for all of us and her sister was fully capable of helping take care of her at this point. I returned rejuvenated and was able to spend a little time with Haley before she had to return home.

One of the many things I learned in that IV room was about NUCCA. It sounded very promising and I felt it was worth looking in to. Maybe this would help with the neurological issues that we just couldn't shake. I called on a Thursday and got an appointment for Monday. NUCCA deals with upper cervical, and after an examination it was evident that Amanda was a mess. She saw her NUCCA doctor twice and was able to stand, taking her first step in one week. We were ecstatic that morning when we showed up for treatment at the West Clinic. We were beaming from ear-to-ear with excitement that we could not contain. We asked to see Dr. J before we did anything else. He came in the room and we told him we had a surprise for him. Amanda stood up and walked! He was ecstatic. She did it for him a second time so he could video it. That day he shared with us that there are times that he sends patients away if he doesn't believe he can help them; he doesn't want to waste their money. He had been at that point with Amanda earlier on. He actually talked to a good friend of his, who happened to be Greg Heister, the very tool God had used back in 2012 to make us aware of the West Clinic in the first place. Thankfully, Greg encouraged him to stick it out a little longer...and we praise God he did. Along with the walking, she was able to read again. She could write, she no longer needed her dark sunglasses, her hearing wasn't as sensitive and her comprehension was normal again. We had a neurological breakthrough! Although NUCCA was an integral part of Amanda being able to walk again, I don't believe it would have been possible without the IV nutritional therapy, as well as all the other treatment under Dr. J's guidance. Her body had to go through internal healing and balancing first to even get to that point.

We decided to go home for Thanksgiving and spend Christmas at home and return in 2015. Amanda and I decided to keep her ability to walk a secret, so as to surprise our family. Dr. J sent two young men back to Florida with us to video this unveiling.

Paul and the other kids were at the airport, along with aunts, uncles, cousins and grandpa. Amanda still didn't have her strength back 100%, so we still used the wheelchair for travel. The plan was to wheel her all the way to our family and then have her stand up and walk.

Oh my word, what an exciting moment that was. There were tears of joy, laughter and sheer amazement among everyone. I'm still surprised myself that we were able to keep it a secret, but it was well worth it. Along with her being able to walk she was now free of her dark sunglasses and wearing regular prescription glasses. She was down to wearing one ear plug. She had gained a little bit of weight, so she didn't look quite so sickly, her smile beamed and she absolutely glowed. She returned like a new person. She had her life back. My kids had their sister back and we had our daughter back. We enjoyed being back together as a family.

Amanda had improved tremendously but there was still need for additional treatment. We returned in February. Amanda, who was now 18, had gotten her driver's license while we were home, was able to stay in Idaho by herself for a while and get around town on her own. I stayed with her for a little bit, then a friend of mine offered to stay with her. I went back to get her right after Easter. I don't think I ever truly thought her health would be restored to this level. I am amazed at how God directed our steps and put such amazing doctors before us, to love and care for Amanda the way they have. I felt as though I was well grounded and strong in my faith in Jesus Christ prior to May 2012. He showed me that my strength comes from Him. On this side of our trial I suppose it's a good thing that I knew the Lord as my personal Savior, otherwise I never would have made it, nor would my marriage have survived. Amanda's sickness was horrible, but the time spent away from my other children while I was in Idaho took its toll on all of us. Even prior to going to Idaho, the way we had allowed sickness to consume our lives was devastating. It hit us hard as adults, and our children even harder. I do have regrets but I can't change anything, I can only seek to make it known to all of my children how important they are, and that I'd do anything in the world for each one of them. They needed us as much as Amanda did. In a way, we had resorted to putting out fires and tending to what was most pressing at the moment. We all suffered because of that.

Upon returning home, Amanda began studying and passed all four parts of her GED the first time. This is pretty incredible, given that she missed her last 3 years of high school. She got a part-time job and has done well. She plans to go to college and work in the medical field. She also plans to visit the West Clinic for continued care and treatment as needed. She feels that she missed out on so much of her youth but she now has her whole life ahead of her to fulfill those dreams.

Amanda wasn't mentally prepared for living the fast-paced lifestyle of a 19-year-old young lady. The type of sickness that she endured hindered her in every way, essentially life stopped for three years. This journey took its toll on her mentally and emotionally as well. With grace and endurance, she will continue to run this race that God has placed before her. We pray for wisdom and grace that comes from the Lord to guide and protect her as well as our other children through these crucial developmental years.

DR. J... DOESN'T CARE WHO GETS THE CREDIT FOR YOU GETTING BETTER HE JUST WANTS YOU TO GET BETTER...

I truly don't know how Dr. J and his team do what they do. They are kind, gracious and patient, and in case you've never noticed, sick people can be very impatient and demanding. Dr. J deals with really, really sick people every day he walks in that office. Many of them are at their wits end. For some, he is their last hope. He was our last hope. He knows the financial hardship of sickness and if he doesn't think he can help you, he certainly doesn't want to take your money. I've heard Dr. J say many times he doesn't care who gets the credit for you getting better, he just wants you to get better...that's me paraphrasing. Dr. J is an amazing man that God has gifted with a brilliant mind and a heart to help others. If you are reading this, please know there is hope. That's something I had to remind myself at times I felt hopeless and my faith wavered. My dose of vitamin H is this:

> We are afflicted in every way, but not crushed; perplexed, but not given to despair; persecuted, but not forsaken; struck down, but not destroyed; always carrying in the body the death of Jesus, so that the life of Jesus may also be manifested in our bodies.   ~2 Corinthians 4:8-10

Take time to renew your minds every day. For me that means spending time in prayer and reading my Bible. It is my source of strength and peace that surpasses all understanding.

3

REASONS WHY
WE GET SICK

THERE ARE A lot of sicknesses in the world that I am not treating, so the reasons why we get sick apply to my patient population and cannot be applied across humanity uniformly. *Hidden Secrets* is a book written for the people afflicted with Lyme disease, chronic fatigue, fibromyalgia, and autoimmune conditions like rheumatoid arthritis, multiple sclerosis, Sjogren's and lupus.

My favorite diseases to treat are of the autoimmune world. Many of my best success stories come from this arena and I challenge the idea that our body is attacking its tissues. I think that the body has a dysfunctional or tricked immune system due to a lingering infection and as the body sends in the cells to address this infection, there is collateral or accidental damage.

For instance, in the case of rheumatoid arthritis, there is uncontrolled inflammation in and around the joint. I believe that the source of this inflammation is an infection in the joint and as the body tries to get rid of the infection, it accidentally damages the surrounding tissues. Why do I think this? Because when you regulate the immune system or make it stronger, patient's symptoms improve and go away. It is my goal when an RA or MS patient walks in the door to give them a million milligrams of vitamin C as fast as possible. If they have true autoimmunity, they should get worse but instead they get better. You can see this in action on our blog: www.dailydosevitaminh.com.

The medical treatment for autoimmune diseases is the exact opposite. Medications that kill the immune system are used. This is not a recipe for long-term health improvement and just some of the effects of this immuno-modulator therapy include gastrointestinal toxicity, stomatitis, alopecia, bone marrow suppression and liver function abnormalities are commonly encountered. The risk factors of getting infections go up substantially. In my opinion giving a medicine that kills the immune system is the opposite of what we should be doing. I enjoy treating the autoimmune spectrum.

Before we can talk about what conditions respond to *Hidden Secrets*, we need to discuss why people get sick. People get sick for the following reasons:

1. Lifestyle choices
2. Magic bullet treatments
3. Emotional conflict
4. Genetics
5. Environmental triggers
6. Wrong doctors, wrong treatments
7. Financial obstacles to treatments

8. Father Time and wearing out

The number one reason people get sick is lifestyle. This is something really important, because patients are always looking for the magic bullet. They're looking for a magic cure. Really the cure is their knife and fork, and second is their sleeping patterns. It's so important to make sure that the patients understand that their lifestyle choices will catch up with them. Sometimes it doesn't catch up with them until their 60's. Sometimes it catches up with them

THE NUMBER ONE REASON PEOPLE GET SICK IS LIFE-STYLE.

in their 20's. Not getting enough sleep, enough water, fulfilling emotional relationships, poor food choices and excessive electromagnetic frequency poisoning are causing chronic illness. Recognizing that you, as the patient, have to change your habits is critical in getting better.

Number two is bad genes. I joke about the bad genes process, but sometimes you get a recessive trait from your mom or dad. Sometimes in homeopathy you get a miasm, which is the environmental opportunity to express a genetic trait. When you are fighting against DNA and then add an environment that causes the illness to flourish, it makes for a harder road to follow. These are hard cases to treat—not impossible but difficult.

George Burns was a comedian who lived to be 100 years old and was very famous. Every time he was interviewed he had a martini or a cigar in his hand. He'd say, "The recipe for health is two cigars and two martinis every day!" Then you hear about the 23-year-old secretary whose boss smokes, she gets second-hand lung cancer and dies. It just doesn't seem fair that you can have someone who's abusing themselves for a century and someone who's trying to live right, but gets sick and catches some difficult disease. I tell everybody, "Welcome to the world of genetics! Some people are made out of Super glue, and some people are made out of Elmer's glue!" Much of what happens is related to our family history, but sometimes it's just a case of genes. Some people get coded for genes where their DNA is literally bulletproof. They go through life abusing themselves, not eating very well, and not having a sleep schedule. They just seem to do everything wrong and nothing seems to faze them!

And then, you have other people that are absolutely committed in every way to their health. They eat perfectly. They get themselves on a schedule, they practice journaling, prayer, meditation and yoga, and they seem to really struggle with their health. Because I'm a very religious person, I think that maybe that is our chore, or our task in life. Some people are given the assignment to deal with health problems for their ecclesiastical trials. It can be tough answering that question. Sometimes people are dealt a bad hand.

Let food be thy medicine and medicine be thy food.

~Hippocrates

This cannot be overstated. You cannot overestimate the effect diet has on health. It's so important that I devote a future chapter on it. We have a saying in the office, "You are what you eat...and if you are what you eat, are you fast, cheap, and easy?" So many times we've made it convenient, and really easy to get foods that taste good but don't have a lot of nutritional value. Just remember that the healthier and more alive your food is, the healthier and more alive you will be. Those patients that are eating clean are much easier to help than those that are eating fast food, microwave dinners, and gas station food.

A frequently overlooked problem for patients is their liquid intake. The American people are so susceptible to being convinced that liquid calories, sport drinks and meal replacers are healthier than quick foods. I am not so sure. This is a chink in a lot of people's armor. Overconsumption of morning coffee, soda pop, energy drinks, green tea, and fruit juice is a major factor in prevention of getting your health back.

Patients ask me all of the time, "what am I supposed to drink?" I reply, "Water." "But Dr. West, I don't like water!" Well, train yourself to like it, or be prepared to either be sick or to spend a lot of money with your doctor.

The other thing that I see tremendous abuse with is sleeping patterns. People don't get the rest that they need. They'll sleep three or four hours and then augment that with a bunch of caffeine in their system such as energy drinks, coffee, soda pop, etc. They're pushing themselves all the time and exhausting their adrenals, and they're literally too tired to sleep! I don't know if anybody has experienced this: you get to the point where you're so tired and then you can't sleep because you literally don't even have enough energy to shut off your systems. It sounds a little bit counterintuitive but sometimes, if you give people just a little bit of energy before they go to bed, they can actually get into rest mode.

While I am not a mind/body doctor, it's important to discuss emotions. I have read many books about the effect of emotions on health. This ranges from an acute pharyngitis to cancer. It's critical to address unresolved emotions. Mind/body therapy is essential to health. When we added this therapy to our treatment plans, we started getting people better—and faster than we had ever done in the past.

We have to identify emotional decompression outlets for patients. That means we have to create a system or activity that the patient handles their emotional conflict. This is done through therapy, counseling, prayer, meditation, deep breathing and my favorite, journaling. Some patients know what the emotional conflict is and others discover it at our clinic.

The biggest suggestion here is to stop comparing yourself to others. Whether it's health, finances, family relationships, cars, money, or success, this emotional baggage of comparing your worst to others' best has to be addressed. Without doing this, treatments will always be limited in their effectiveness. This is particularly important for spousal relationships. Patients will say, "Well, how come my spouse isn't sick?" They aren't asking because they want their spouse to be sick, they are asking to try and figure out how people can be in the same environment and yet one is sick and one is healthy.

...STOP COMPARING YOURSELF TO OTHERS.

There are many reasons. For example: there are genetic differences at play. Some people just have incredibly strong DNA and some don't. Some spouses don't have the emotional upheaval and burden that the sick spouse has. It is helpful to have emotional outlets and sometimes counseling therapy is also an important consideration in the healing process.

I am not sure of the percentages but I am not surprised when many of my patients with debilitating sickness confide in me that they are the victim of emotional, physical or sexual abuse. Many patients bury, hide and suppress these terrible experiences, and I don't think their physiology can handle that much emotional conflict. It manifests itself in illness. I am not suggesting that all chronic illness patients are the victims of abuse, but I see it more often than not.

Here's an example. Let's call this patient "Mary". Mary had been sick for decades. She was able to function but life was a chore. She heard that we had some favorable outcomes for her disease. I will talk about the mistake health care providers make when we treat disease instead of the individual. We started a treatment program for Mary. We made fantastic progress until about the 50% mark and then we just plateaued. No matter what we did, we just couldn't seem to help her improve any more than 50%. Naturally, I want every patient to be 100% better. I am an optimist.

During one visit, I asked her if there were any unresolved emotions that could be the obstacle to healing. There was a long and uncomfortable pause. I was worried that I had ventured into territory that I was not invited. She told me that she had been abused by a family member and had never recovered. While I was expecting something like this, what she said next was surprising. "I think I can get through this, but I don't know if my husband will." I told her that most spouses underestimate the love capacity of their mates. But that wasn't what she meant. "I know that my husband loves me more than life itself, I have never told him, not because he wouldn't accept me, but because I worry that the family member that hurt me would cease to exist. My husband might end up in prison and that is why I haven't told anyone for 28 years." Both wife and husband were able to get therapy and after the emotional hurdle was addressed, the patient once again had a huge positive response to treatment.

When I talk about environmental triggers, it does encompass food, liquid intake and relationships but I am specifically meaning your living surroundings. So many people are in black mold environments, heavy metal environment, sound pollution, chemical laden surroundings of agriculture, pet pollution, and electromagnetic frequency (EMF) toxicity.

It makes sense that you don't want a black wall of mold or lead-based paint, or to live next to the airport runway or on top of a train track, but I do want to talk more about pets and EMF. I am all about pets but how many pet owners will take their pet into the vet periodically to be de-wormed and then don't get de-wormed themselves? Then I learn later that the patient is sleeping with the pet, kissing the pet, or sharing food off the same plate. Hey, I am not going to say you can't have pets, but if you are kissing your cat, licking your dog or smooching your horse, you need to stop. And if you are having your pet sleep in your bed, I strongly suspect you have parasites. Both you and your pet need to be treated with a parasite formula. EMF causes a lot of people to be sick. We are electrical beings and when we put ourselves in an electrical field, near LED lights, or have constant cell phone usage, I think it has an effect on us. When people get a health sanctuary that is free of EMF, their physiology responds.

I will say repeatedly that the health care environment is full of great people but the system is evil. Wrong doctors giving the wrong treatments cause people to be sick. Our system is backwards. We subsidize prescriptive interventions and surgery while financially penalizing people that want to do lifestyle, nutrition, and non-prescriptive therapies and treatments first. We should be doing the least costly, least invasive procedures first and then if those don't help people we should move to drugs and surgery. We have it backward; we jump right to the most expensive and most invasive system first. If you go to a surgeon, his training is to fix you with surgery. If you go to an internist, his training is to treat you with Rx.

Unfortunately, in the United States of America, if you have the resources to get better, you'll have a much better chance of getting true health care help. Managing symptoms is what is happening, but they aren't fixing the cause. We have effective ways to treat pain but if we aren't careful we end up with zombies and addicts. Not having the financial resources to pursue the treatment best suited to help you, causes emotional conflict and interferes with your ability to get better.

The last reason why we get sick is Father Time. This is the hardest truth to accept as a health care provider. No matter how hard we try, you can't win the battle that we are eventually going to wear out. While my religious beliefs do not accept that this life is the end of our spirit or our soul, I do accept that there is an end for all of us. Sometimes it is 20; others it is 85. When God decides it's time for you to go, you are going. I thought this applied to everyone else but believed I could help my father recover from a terminal diagnosis. My father passed away at 79 years old after a bout of ulcerative colitis and hepatorenal syndrome.

WHEN GOD DECIDES IT'S TIME FOR YOU TO GO, YOU ARE GOING.

The magic bullet treatments are what happens when consumers are lulled into a false sense of security that the American health care system has the treatments or is on the verge of discovering a treatment that is going to nullify the consequences of lifestyle choice. This doesn't apply to the small percentage of people that strive to do everything right through diet, exercise, and yet still are afflicted by illness. This applies to many patients that just don't think that hard living is going to catch up to them. While not wanting to be harsh, I have to practice tough love here...There is no magic pill for disease. There is no magic surgery for decades of ignoring your health. This is the most important component of understanding why people get sick. I do not believe there is one single magic bullet or treatment for chronic disease.

The reason why we get sick, in most instances, is because we've deviated from physical law. Those with religious influence in their life recognize that when we deviate from spiritual law, we are told that this is a sin. What is the treatment for a sin? The repentance process. The word repent comes from the Greek word root "to change," or in other words stop what you are doing and get back on the straight and narrow. Deviation from the laws of health is a symptom. Just like spiritual repentance, we need to have a physical repentance and change. When we abuse physical laws, and we don't sleep, and we're putting junk into our system, we get a symptom! If we want to get rid of that symptom we literally have to do the same thing. We have to repent, or change, from that lifestyle habit that's causing the symptom. That's why if we can get people to change, amazing outcomes often happen. But there has to be the change within the patient.

I follow this axiom, "the more education and information you give to people, the better equipped they are to change." When they come into the office, no matter how good treatments are from other doctors and myself, we can't make long-lasting improvements to their health unless they repent and change lifestyle.

4

THE PROBLEM
WITH SICKNESS CARE
– OUR CURRENT SYSTEM

OUR CURRENT HEALTH care system is a mess. It makes getting healthy harder. It causes emotional barriers, conflict and frustration on the side of patients, mountains of documentation, paperwork, regulations and equal frustration on the health provider side.

I know how to fix my side of the equation but it doesn't work for all patients, only some. I decided in 2009 to get out of the insurance system. My responsibility is not to the insurance carrier or third party administrator, it is to the patient. When you are beholden to no one besides the patient, I believe a level of clarity for the patient's condition is reached that is not reached in the insurance world. However, I feel badly for patients that do not have the option to pay cash for health care services or are in a position to use a flex plan, cafeteria plan, health savings account or health reimbursement arrangement. I also share in this frustration on the consumer side because I have insurance for emergencies and pay thousands of dollars a year for services that I am not going to use.

If you ask people "what's wrong with healthcare?" patients will tell you it's expensive, it's confusing and broken. The health care community will tell you that there is too much paperwork, too much bureaucracy, and not enough money for the time commitment. The insurance community will tell you it's the rising costs of premiums, overly high doctor costs and expensive litigation.

There is some truth to all of the responses. The first thing is that we have a really unusually evil industry. There are some fantastic people in the healthcare industry. I really believe that, almost all doctors have the intention of helping people. It's no one's intention to make people worse, but the industry itself is evil. The reason why it's evil is because there's massive confusion and misinformation. We'll compare running a business to the way we run healthcare. Say you have a car dealership. Someone comes in and tells you, "I want a car." You say, "Great! This is what we're going to do. We'll decide what color and what kind of car we give you. Go home and we'll deliver the car to you. Then, we're going to send you bills"... plural!

We just had this happen with my son. He had a motorcycle accident where he needed stitches, and we took him in to the emergency room. The emergency room people were fantastic. They put him at ease, they were able to take him out of pain and discomfort, and then they called the plastic surgeon. The plastic surgeon came in and he was amazing. He stitched my son back together. Then as we went to check out they said, "Hey, we're going to bill your insurance, and then you pay the deductible or any payment." We have a catastrophic plan with a $10,000.00 deductible. As we started getting bills, my wife would call them up and say, "All right, we're just going to pay this instead of trying to run it through the system. Is there a cash discount?" We've learned that a lot of time you can get a significant discount if you'll pay cash immediately. We tried to pay our bill every single time. We got one bill from the hospital, and then another from the anesthesiologist, and then the plastic surgeon. It seemed like every couple of weeks we were getting a separate bill. I'm thinking, "Man, I thought we had paid this!"

It's antiquated. During the World War II era, people were provided for with a benefit system that got around some wage and compensation laws. That system has continued. We don't know what we're paying for. I really believe that the clearer you are with financial expectations, the better it helps people to heal. Gone are the days, except for some of the specialists or clinics, where you can go in to a medical office and pay cash. Part of the

YOU DON'T KNOW IF THIS IS THE $0.50 ASPIRIN, OR IF THIS IS THE $500.00 ASPIRIN!

problem is that the system is so confusing! We have an insurance component, a government component, we've got situations where you go in, get a service and you don't know what it is going to cost. You don't know if this is the $0.50 aspirin, or if this is the $500.00 aspirin!

I always try and get to the clinic about an hour before we start with patients. One day, about 7:00 a.m., I arrived and there was a patient sitting on the steps with a paper in her hand and she was crying. I opened up the office, and went out to talk to her. She was really sick with an autoimmune condition and we were treating her with vitamin infusions. We can talk about autoimmune in the conditions chapter. Back to the story. She was responding well to the treatment. She had come to the office that day because she was unhappy with what was happening in the medical realm.

I asked her, "I thought you were doing really well. Why are you crying?" She said, "Well, Dr. J, I just got my bill from the hospital. I went in to get a treatment. No one told me what it was going to be, how much it was going to cost, and I have a high insurance deductible!" This was about a month before we started treating her, and they did a special IgG antibody treatment with one IV. Her bill for that single IV in the hospital was $42,000.00! She said, "I got no help from that IV whatsoever! I have been at the West Clinic for five weeks for treatments and I have spent $1,100.00, and I'm doing so much better! How come no one told me my options at the hospital?"

I FELT LIKE I WAS TREATING THE INSURANCE COMPANY AND NOT THE PATIENT!

When we go into the healthcare arena, the first problem is confusion. The second problem we have is we've advocated patient responsibility to a third-party payer. When the clinic was billing insurance, people would say, "Well, bill my insurance, and I will pay the balance." Many times the insurance is dictating the care for the patient. I call it compensation slavery! The doctors say, "Well, I'm only going to do what insurances pay!" And then insurance is saying, "Well, we're only going to pay for this," or "We're only going to pay for that," or "You need to get preauthorization!" This is one of the biggest reasons why we got out of billing insurance. I felt like I was treating the insurance company and not the patient! We had to have a paradigm shift. When people come into the office, our responsibility is to the patient, not the insurance company.

That has really shielded patients from the true cost of things. Obviously, when we talk about healthcare, there's always the concern about litigation and legal expenses. If you don't do something as a healthcare provider are you going to get sued because you didn't follow the reasonable standards for care? If someone comes in for a headache, the likelihood of them having a brain tumor, by percentages, has got to be really, really small. But if we don't do a CT scan and an MRI and a full workup, we think, "Should we have done that?" I think a lot of decisions, particularly in the traditional medical world, are based on covering your A-S-S!

The other concern is the direct marketing of electrician's tape to put over the oil light, which is the pharmaceutical advertising. Let's pretend you are going down the road and you occasionally glance at your dashboard to make sure you are following the speed limit and that your vehicle is running correctly. One time you look down and you see the oil light is on. The current medical system solution to that is to hand you a piece of black electrician's tape and say put this over the oil light and then you won't notice it. Common sense tells us that we are eventually going to end up with an overhaul but that's what many doctors in the medical world do with many of the prescriptive medicine interventions. I am joking but also serious when I say this.

Why don't we figure out what is wrong with the engine before we start giving pain killers, steroids, and happy pills? In many instances, they are not fixing the problem, they are hiding it. Think about a traditional office visit. They tell you what you have and tell you to go to your doctor and ask for a prescription(s). Take two of these and call me tomorrow. 60% of Americans are taking prescriptive medications and most of them are taking more than one.

One of the things that we do in the clinic is we print out the side effects for medications from a Physicians Desk Reference and review it with the patients. Many times it's a struggle to identify which symptoms are abnormal physiology or the disease process and which symptoms are the side effects of the medication given to the patient. I am not anti-medicine or anti-pharmaceutical, I'm just really, really cautious when it comes to aggressive interventions. I want to have people take responsibility for their health. With the current system, it makes it harder for people to take that responsibility.

We've talked about drugs already. The other thing is this: if you go to a guy with a hammer in his hand, everything looks like a nail. When people have aches and pains or a musculoskeletal problem, they'll go in to the orthopedic surgeon. The orthopedic surgeon will ask, "How can I fix you with surgery?" It's not that he is a bad person or he's anxious to do surgery, but that's the way he was trained. If you go to someone that isn't a surgeon, he asks, "How can I fix you without surgery?" One of the problems in healthcare is that you almost have to be a doctor to know which doctor you should go to! If it's above the diaphragm, you go see an internal medicine guy. If it's below the diaphragm, you go see a gastroenterologist. If it's a liver problem, you go see a liver doctor. If it's a kidney problem, you see the nephrologist. If it's lower down from the kidneys, you see a urologist. If it's a female urinary problem, maybe you see a gynecologist. One of the difficulties is that we've

ONE OF THE PROBLEMS IN HEALTHCARE IS THAT YOU ALMOST HAVE TO BE A DOCTOR TO KNOW WHICH DOCTOR YOU SHOULD GO TO!

segmented everybody into the subspecialties. We sometimes lose sight of the big picture. I've had so many patients that have come in and have said, "I have a healthcare problem!" There were some cardiovascular concerns and they went to see the cardiologist. They said he asked them how they felt and they told him. He said, "No, no, no! I only deal with your heart! With your other concerns, you've got to go see a different doctor for that! I only do the heart!"

Sometimes people go to the wrong specialist. They are slated for surgery when perhaps there is a least aggressive or lesser expensive procedure. I tell my patients that our goal is to do the least expensive, least aggressive intervention first. If that doesn't work, then we go to the next step. And we continue on until something works. Again, I'm not anti-medicine, but I think that doctors are doing a lot of aggressive medicine that doesn't need to be done, they are not educated about integrative or alternative interventions. Part of the reason is that the system is set up so that doctors get heavily influenced by the drugs and surgical equipment industry. Just follow the money trail.

The system actually pushes people into the most expensive system first. I frequently say, "If there was a level playing field, and if patients could have the opportunity to choose whatever intervention they could, I think we would really cut down a lot on the surgical and expensive interventions." The reason they got used so much is because that is what's paid for! We've shielded the patient from accountability, we subsidized the most expensive treatments, and we have a lot of advertising for aggressive and expensive medications. Those are the big problems. You've never seen anybody on TV saying, "Hey, take vitamin D3, it really helps with your hormones." Or, "Take vitamin C, it's really good for your colds or connective tissue."

Pharmaceutical companies are in business to make a profit just like everybody else and they make drugs for profit. They have the research and development, and they want to recoup their cost and make a ton of money.

Most of the time, the pharmaceutical companies are taking something that's natural (and you can't patent a natural substance), they're tweaking that molecule and making it synthetic. Then, they take it to market.

The reason why the West Clinic has such a fantastic patient base is because we became a cash-based clinic. We are asking the patient to pay us for the services that are rendered. I don't have the patients that are looking for an easy out, insurance reimbursement or doctor shopping. Yes, it is unfortunate that people pay into an insurance system where they can't get the type of care they want. I am one of those, I pay insurance for a system that I don't use, but I have catastrophic coverage.

The patients that come to the West Clinic are really committed to their healthcare. But healthcare, overall, has to put the accountability back on the patient. From the patient's perspective, the more they're educated and the more they understand about their conditions, the better their compliance is.

I made this mistake early on in my career. I was learning about all these supplements, biochemistry pathways, and everything else. People would come into the office, and I'd say, "Okay, you take this supplement for this condition and this supplement for this condition and this mineral for hair and this vitamin for this and this herb for this!"

People were walking out of the clinic with 25 bottles of supplements and I was thinking that I was such a good doctor because I had given them a supplement for every pathway, deficiency, symptom and disease. It didn't work. They would be so overwhelmed that they would go home and put their pills in the cupboard. I would see them six months later and they would say, "Dr. J, I have the same problem!" I would ask, "what about taking this herb and this vitamin and this mineral?" They'd reply, "Oh, I still have it!" I'm thinking, *No, no! That was a 30-day supply! You shouldn't have that!* What I'd learned was that the least number of things that I prescribed to people, the better their compliance was.

The compliance of the patient following the recommendations goes up even further if the patient is provided a printout sheet that says, "This is why you need this vitamin. This is why you need this mineral. For example, magnesium helps with muscle cramps! Vitamin D helps with your immune system and hormones!"

If I've given them a written printout, they can read it and they'll understand why they need the supplements. Then their compliance goes way off the charts. When people are given the least amount of supplements, they are usually more compliant.

I want to give people enough information so that they make a change. I give them lifestyle parameters so they can make wise choices in their diet and daily schedules.

Thoughts on Medical Doctors

Patients ask me my thoughts on medical doctors. With any profession there are good guys and bad guys. I believe nearly every doctor genuinely wants people to improve and get better but it's the system that is bad. So many times medical doctors are taught that prescription drug therapy is the only way forward.

My frustration with the medical system is that MDs receive different training and are limited by the standards of care to what treatments they can provide. Most do not provide services like nutritional therapy, chiropractic therapy, neural prolotherapy, neural therapy, vitamin infusion therapy and oxidative medicine.

We all get trained in our respective fields, so to the guy with the hammer in his hand, everything looks like a nail. If you go to a surgeon, it's natural for him to say, "How can I fix you with surgery?" If you go to an internal medicine doctor, "How can I fix you with a prescription?" If you come to my clinic, you'll get everything but drugs and surgery first. Again, I am not anti-medicine by any means but I want to exhaust the other pathways first.

The industry is broken, many times it twists and contorts the true intent of the doctor by all of the regulations, insurance, pre-authorization and compensation slavery (insurance dictating your treatment options). I know a lot of medical doctors that are awesome people and really want to help people; it's a shame that our system really seems to prevent that.

5

BARRIERS TO HEALING

WHY DO SOME people get better and some don't? Welcome to the world of the art and practice of being a healer. I have seen a lot of patients that were very ill who I didn't think could be helped. But they turned around and got better. While others who I thought would be easy fixes didn't respond or they even got worse and continued on down the road of ill health. Why? What is the common denominator in getting better or getting worse? There are so many factors that are at play in health and disease. Some people are going to get better because they are doing everything right and they just need a tune-up from their doctor. Others are going to get better because they get an overhaul. Some patients don't want to get better. Some people are prevented from getting better because they do not have a support system. Some patients like the attention and focus from being sick. Some people can't get better because their body has forgotten what it is like to be healthy. The neat thing is when people understand the barriers to healing entirely new levels of improvement are possible. I've mentioned these barriers in Chapter 3: Why We Get Sick.

You must be willing to change. By following simple rules the body has the amazing ability to respond. Once those rules are in place, I love the frequent feedback from patients, "I didn't know I could feel so good!" If you don't change, you are always going to struggle with your health. We will go over the rules of health in chapter 14.

The Wrong Doctors, Treatments and Treatment Plan

So many people get the wrong treatment for their condition. Just because everyone is doing it, doesn't make it the best way to treat the condition. From a health care perspective, I get so frustrated with the pharmaceutical influence on health care but from a business perspective I grudgingly admire them. They get a lot of people on their product and then keep them there for life. There are numerous symptoms and diseases I could use here for examples. High blood pressure, allergies, diabetes, arthritis, and cholesterol management are just some of the things that are so much more effectively treated than by the mainstream medical system.

How do you know you are getting the wrong treatment? Ask yourself and listen to your intuition. Is the current treatment plan getting me to where I want to go?

Ask yourself if you like the plan, the side-effects or the risk factors. How do I feel when I am following the treatment recommendations? If any of these don't feel right, then there is your answer. I invite you to explore the many different options to your health care concern. The third barrier to healing is disease progression. If patients wait too long before changing their lifestyle, food intake, medical nutritional therapy, rehabilitation, exercise and mind/body healing, you can't reverse the effects on the body. I have seen this happen many times in rheumatoid arthritis. Once the joint has started to deform, you can still help with the inflammation, redness, swelling and function but you can never make that joint normal. You want to get the treatments before the disease leaves irreversible damage to the body.

The fourth barrier to healing is the most complex. Some people do not want to get better, either by choice or subconsciously. If you are the majority of people that truly want to get better, please don't get offended, but do be aware that you may be inadvertently sabotaging yourself. Other times, especially with terminal disease, the patient is suffering through the treatments to appease family members and loved ones, not because they really want the treatment or even believe that the treatment is going to work. I see this a lot in terminal patients. As an alternative medicine provider, I never thought I was going to be involved in end-of-life discussions, but it happens regularly. Patients have been through the medical system, chemotherapy, radiation, surgery and despite the best efforts of their medical team, the treatments didn't work. Then the patient comes to my office and asks what alternatives are available. Sometimes there isn't a viable solution to restore their health, but I know we can help those patients with their quality of life.

ONE OF THE MOST IMPORTANT QUESTIONS DOCTORS SHOULD ASK PATIENTS IS, "DO YOU WANT TO GET BETTER??

One of the most important questions doctors should ask patients is, "Do you want to get better?" When you know what the patient really wants, you can design your treatment plan to fit the patient's expectations. My terminal patients often say, "I want you to help me be as healthy as possible before I die." Others say, "I am only here because my husband, son, or friend insisted I be here."

Many patients do not want to get better and they know it and live it. Others don't want to get better and don't even know it. There are patients that do not want to get better because they enjoy the love, attention and focus they get from being ill.

This ranges from mild behavior to mental and emotional abuse to the caregiver. The patient is not trying to deliberately make their support circle or care giver miserable. The patient needs help and they are trying to communicate that but they don't know how, so they use physical symptoms as non-verbal communication. Almost always there is unresolved emotional conflict that has caused the patient to act this way. This is commonly observed in the office when the caregiver leaves and the patient acts one way and then when the caregiver returns the patient ratchets up the attention factor. These cases respond very well to mind/body healing in conjunction with physical healing. Other patients do not want to get better because of self-esteem, personal accountability, and excuse mindset. I hear this consistently, "If I didn't have [disease], I could have, should have or would have been this or done that." I could have been an astronaut, but because of the [disease], I am regulated to being a sick person! When you start balancing their physiology, clean up their lifestyle, and get the patient to do everything they are supposed to do, you'll discover this possible problem when you do a re-evaluation.

The system in our clinic is that we perform our initial assessment and new patient workup, then provide a treatment recommendation with a calendar and financial parameters. During every visit we have the patient fill out a daily update sheet. On the sheet it asks the patient from the time of the treatment until now if they are better, the same or different? Then there is a space on the form to ask the doctor questions.

The patient will say that they are 10%, then 25%, then 30% better in their own handwriting and then when we do the re-evaluation on the 10th visit, the patient will say, "I am not any better. I am just not improving." This is exactly opposite of what they have filled out every day.

So what's happening? The patient is in very uncomfortable territory. Since the symptoms are going away, the patient realizes that they can no longer blame their sickness for their set of circumstances and now they are in a position that they have to accept responsibility for no longer blaming their illness. It can be a very hard transition. Mind/body therapy is essential in these cases.

Others have emotional conflict and baggage and do not feel they are worthy of being healthy or having a happy life. It's almost like they are punishing themselves for a past mistake, deviation from parental values, a divorce, a death of a loved one or some other experience that has left the patient scarred. My experience is that most patients want to get better and I feel bad for those that are going through versions of self-sabotage. There can be versions of conscious/subconscious barriers to healing. For those reading this book because someone close to you is sick, be aware of this. Sometimes you will need therapy to not unconsciously be an enabler in addition to the treatments needed for the patient.

An enormous barrier to healing is the inner circle. This door swings both ways. It can help facilitate a miraculous turnaround or it can be the mire that does not allow the patient to be healthy. It can be a conscious or subconscious barrier. Relationships are critical for healing, to the extent that you can have healthy and fulfilling relationships in your life. Your response to treatment will be better if you do.

By the way, if you know anyone with perfect relationships in their life, you don't know them well enough. No one has perfect relationships, is stress free, or has the perfect life. The admonition here is that we should try our best but do not expect a life without conflict. Just like the patient that gets attention from being sick, certain caregivers enjoy the attention, notoriety and validation from being the lifesaver for the patient. "That husband is so devoted to his sick wife, that's amazing!" or "I can't believe so and so stays married to her husband. He is always sick and needs her help. She's a saint and is going to heaven." I don't know if this is a conscious decision but I have seen the caregiver be uncomfortable with the patient's improvement and less dependency.

The flip side is more likely. This is when the inner support circle opposes or is passive aggressive and does not support the patient treatment decision. This has a devastating effect on the patient. You may not believe or support the treatments the patient decides to do, but you can absolutely affect the treatments by your actions. Please do not be a barrier. Do not underestimate how much contribution or detriment the inner circle has on a patient case. The impact is enormous.

Let me see if I can explain how I do it. After being in the trenches for 16 years, I have more latitude than I used to; my tolerance is much improved. I get asked daily about common and uncommon treatments. At one time, I used to be very outspoken on certain therapies and if I didn't recognize the therapy I was asked about, I would outright dismiss or impugn the therapy. Well, just like a teenager that knows everything, once you get a little life experience you start to understand that your viewpoint and biasness towards the unknown may not be accurate. I accept therapies that help the patient.

This means that I don't have to understand the therapy to be open to it. I ask the patient, "Do you perceive a benefit from trying XYZ?" If they say yes my response is that you should keep doing it. If there is no perceived benefit or if the treatment is causing unwanted side-effects, then we need to explore other avenues.

My goal is to get the patient better. I don't care who gets the credit, what treatments they do, or where they go as long as they get better. My charge is to help the patient along that journey, not to be an egotistical or arrogant doctor that might prevent the incorporation of a valuable healing intervention.

Periodically, I'll get asked if the treatment in question is all placebo and my response is "does it matter?" If you think that meditation is helping your condition or meditation is a placebo and you start to feel better, all that matters is you are doing better. Who cares if it is placebo, as long as it's working you have started your health care journey.

The last barrier to healing is a fact of life and that is financial. Unfortunately, if people cannot afford treatments, they will not get better. Many of the treatments necessary to "cure" a condition are not covered by insurance—lifestyle, exercise, vitamin infusions, medical nutritional therapy, mind/body healing. If patients can't afford the treatments, they won't get better, it's a grim reality. We'll talk more about the financial investment in health in chapter 14.

6

THE DIFFERENCE MAKER

DURING ALMOST EVERY patient interview (the most important part of the healing process), I will get asked why we are different. "Dr. West, what makes you think you can help me when the other doctors or clinics have failed? Why do you think you can help me?"

While I wish I could say I have helped every person, that is not correct. Sometimes, what I have to offer may not be what the patient needs. But we will always recommend them to a doctor or another clinic. Still, I am always surprised when we can't at least make an improvement in the patient's life, if not an improvement in their condition. I genuinely expect every patient to have an improvement and even in terminal cases a better quality of life before they move on to the next phase (I don't believe this is the end of our existence).

What medicine loves is cookbook medicine. You name it, blame it, and then contain it. One diagnosis, one disease and one treatment. Same medicine, same procedure, and same dosage. The problem with much of medicine is that we've trained a generation of doctors who haven't been taught to think.

~ Henry West

Frequently, I sit with patients, hear their story and ask, "What is the medical treatment plan or recommendations?" Sometimes it is logical, sometimes unusual and sometimes illogical. Nothing surprises me. Just recently, I had a college athlete with a chronic painful toe. After a series of treatments, physical therapy, orthotics and prescriptive therapy, the doctors' recommendation was "let's cut off your toe." We had a great outcome using regenerative injection therapy, neural therapy and nutritional building block therapy for the nerve.

THE BIGGEST DIFFERENCE BETWEEN WHAT I PRACTICE AND WHAT IS OFFERED IN TRADITIONAL MEDICINE IS THAT YOU MUST TREAT EACH PATIENT AS AN INDIVIDUAL.

The biggest difference between what I practice and what is offered in traditional medicine is that you must treat each patient as an individual. There is no protocol for Lyme disease, blood pressure, arthritis, or chronic fatigue. It goes back to this—the most important vitamin or mineral is the one the patient needs, not a pre-set protocol.

I was asked to write a chapter in the *Difference Maker* series and after I wrote the chapter, I realized that it was a great fit for this book too. Here is why I believe I can make a difference. I was sitting in my chair in the clinic, listening intently to another tragic health care story. The patient was telling me of her travel through the health care world and her complicated set of symptoms. First was the onset, then the emotional toll, the physical toll and then the financial toll. Because she didn't fit into a specific diagnostic category, she had some symptoms of multiple sclerosis, but not all; some symptoms of fibromyalgia, but not all; she inevitably ended up in the "it's not us, it's you" medical category of it's all in your head. "Here, take this happy pill (antidepressant) and call me in a couple of months." This is typically what her medical person told her. But despite seeing 11 medical specialists, no one had ever tried to listen to what happens on a normal day, what she was eating/drinking and not one doctor had tried to restore function by balancing her physiology.

When I heard another story of mismanagement of a lost and sick soul, I couldn't help but think, "Nothing is ever going to surprise me! I have heard it all." I just wanted to tell this patient and every other one, "Yes, I can help you!" I may not cure you. I may not take away all of your infirmities, but I really believe I can improve your quality of life. Vitamin infusion therapy, detoxification, adjustments, oxidative medicine and specific vitamin/mineral therapy help with nearly everyone. Couple that with the basics of good food, good air, good water, put the body on a schedule and then get very specific on giving the body the right bio-mechanic correction, hormone balancing and working on the emotional stresses and you now have a recipe that helps nearly all conditions.

You see, I had just had an amazing clinical experience. The one that makes you feel like if your professional life was to stop right there, you would know that you really helped at least one person, one family and one generation. It is my goal to get at least one amazing video testimonial every day and I was on a roll.

I have had a patient tell me that she had come to my office to die and not only was she alive, she was thriving! She went from death's door to enrolling in a health care program, because I had helped her. I was riding the healer's high. I thought that after 16 years in the trenches and 10,000 new patient interviews, I had heard it all. This was not true. I am constantly surprised by what patients tell me about their experience prior to coming to the clinic. Here are the more common responses from medical doctors to patients who have a chronic disease or condition:

- It's all in your head.
- You just want attention.
- You need to get off the internet, because it will convince you that you have a disease that you don't have.
- Just get a job.
- Quit being a hypochondriac
- You just need a happy pill
- You need to have an orgasm
- Just take this Rx for life.
- Just taking a pill might make you feel better. The pill doesn't matter.
- You have a disease that we don't know about.
- If you Google this condition and find something out, please tell me.

I have amazing clinical outcomes from people with chronic conditions. Chapter 9 tells the story behind the story.

I was bustling down the hall with my assistant in tow. I love having a busy office and today was no different. I love being so busy that I don't have time to sit down. I just go from patient to patient until after 5 p.m. and then go home, rinse, dry and repeat.

My patient, Greg, stands in front of me in the hall. He puts up a great big hand like a police officer at an intersection and says, "Dr.

West, stop right there." Uh oh. I'm thinking "what happened?" My mind starts asking, what's wrong? All of my patients are really important to me and I get really concerned when I think there is a problem.

Greg had come to the office at the recommendation of a famous retired NBA athlete, John Stockton. Greg had been diagnosed with reactive arthritis and was put on some very powerful but very toxic immuno-modulator (translation: chemotherapy) medications before coming to my office. Greg was not doing well and the retired athlete had told him to drop everything and get to my office.

Naturally, Greg was skeptical because who would live and practice in Pocatello, Idaho? Then John told him, "Greg, I can go anywhere in the world for health care and this is where I would go. Just get in the car and go there."

About a year before, Greg had limped and walked into the office as a very sick, very tired and very skeptical patient. His background was as an investigative journalist (he has 15 Emmys) and if I had known that, I always tell Greg, I would have never let him come to the office. He couldn't move well, his stomach was horrible with severe bowel problems; his circulation was terrible, with brain fog, depression, anxiety and everything in between. During the course of the treatment, Greg got his hope and his health back and his keen investigative sense. I was in for the experience of a lifetime, and I thought I had experienced every patient interaction available in my world. You see, Greg is one of my wonderful patient outcome miracles. He has completely beat reactive arthritis (it was misdiagnosed). It was really chronic Lyme disease. His story on its own is miraculous. We treated him with IV Vitamin C, ozone, lifestyle modifications (he started eating better and taking care of himself), and specific vitamin therapy. He was a walking billboard for tough cases.

"Dr. West, you gotta let me talk to some of the patients!" Talk to patients? What's Greg asking now? I thought, *All he does is talk to people.* He was always social in the patient treatment areas. He said, "I have my video camera and I want your permission to interview patients on camera." *Well, who wants to go to a doctor's office and be videotaped* was the immediate thought in my mind. How are our patients going to take a great big investigative reporter (Greg is 6'6") with a video camera going around my office?

Every once in a while, you have one of those moments when the universe stops because of a profound revelation. I was happy in my own little cocoon (in my integrative medical practice) and didn't realize all of the miracles that were happening on a daily basis.

You see, I expect to help everyone that receives treatment at the clinic (maybe they will not be completely cured, but I believe that we will improve our patient's health and their quality of life). Greg tells me, "I want to document the miracles I see at the clinic."

I was so absorbed by patient care that I wasn't completely aware of the impact of my life's work, until Greg started walking around the office with his video camera.

One of the greatest feelings of happiness in my life is to see the impact of working with patients on a daily basis. Sometimes we take for granted what blessing we are to patients and what Greg did by videotaping these patients is special. Here are two of the hundreds of patient testimonials and stories that are really important: www.dailydosevitaminh.com.

7

SOLUTIONS

NOW THAT WE have identified the problem, are aware of barriers to healing and you have found the right doctor, it's time to get to work. Let me introduce you to the most important part of your treatment team, you! Take a moment and perform a self-evaluation on how you are treating yourself. If your body was a machine, would it keep running? Do you run it full-speed near RPM red line at nonstop intervals? Do you change the oil? Do you put in the best fuel? Do you wash it and put it away?

Solutions:

1. Evaluate yourself.
2. Take responsibility for your health.
3. Change your lifestyle.
4. Find the doctor that you like and is compatible with you.
5. Take control.
6. Receive the appropriate treatments.

It's really funny for both of us when the patient says, "I eat really, really well!" I'll ask him, "How do you treat your body?" "I eat really well! I take really good care of myself!" I'll go through the daily review, and they'll say, "Well, I get up in the morning, and I have a granola bar. And then I go to lunch with my coworkers. I'll have some lasagna or some casserole at night. I may have a yogurt or some ice cream before I go to bed." And then, I repeat it back to them, and they say, "Wow! That sounds awful! I thought I was doing a lot better!" I don't hear about them eating any green things. I don't hear any vegetables. The solution is to empower people and remind them that you are what you eat! You are also what you absorb.

It's not surprising if you realize how you treat your body. You would never treat a piece of equipment that way. It's time to take ownership and start working on yourself. I would recommend doing a daily review:

• What time do you go to bed?
• How long does it take to get to sleep?
• Do you sleep through the night? Why not?
• What time do you get up?
• When are you first eating? Preferably breakfast.
• When are you eating again? Preferably lunch.
• When are you eating again after that? Preferably dinner.
• Are you having any snacks? What kind of snacks?
• Do you eat before bed?
• What is your liquid intake?
• Do you take supplements? If you do, do you notice a difference by taking them?
• Do you take Rx medications? If you do, have you asked your doctor if it is possible to get off of them?

I see so many problems that are improved simply by just getting enough water into people's systems. There's a fantastic book called *You're Not Tired, You're Toxic!* There's another one called *Your Body's Many Cries for Water!* I tell people, "We've got to make sure that you're getting enough water!" People will sometimes say, "Well, I don't like water!" I'll tell them, "Well, it's a free country. You can have your symptoms as long as you want! But if you want to get better, you need to increase your water intake."

The first thing is to remind people that there are no shortcuts in how they treat themselves. We get one really nice piece of equipment for our life. We get one Ferrari! And some people do a really good job with that Ferrari. They're always changing the oil, they're putting the best fuel in it, and they're putting it into a garage at night. Other people take that Ferrari up into the mountains and go four-wheeling, and they never change the oil, they never wash it. Then they wonder, "How come my car isn't running the way that it used to?" That's one of the solutions—drink enough water.

The other solution is figuring out what is wrong, because something happened with someone's physiology to have them have an acute or chronic condition. Is it in a lifestyle, is it trauma, and is it autosuggestion? So many times people turn into self-fulfilling prophecies! I'm not a mind/body healer, but I recognize that the mind and the body are really intricately connected. You can't treat the body without the mind and the mind without the body! There's such a strong emotional component to fibromyalgia. We can ask the question, "Are you depressed because you hurt, or because you're hurt does it make you depressed?" Giving people the right tools for their mind-body healing is really important. Finding out and making sure that people aren't having autosuggestion is so important. I've had people come into the office and say, "I know I'm sick! I'm going to be sick! I'm always going to be sick!"

You know what? When you keep telling yourself that you are going to be sick, you will be sick.

I had a patient like this about five years ago. They came into the office and said, "Dr. West, I want to know if I have cancer, and is there anything that I can do to prevent it?" I'm an alternative medicine provider; I'm not a cancer specialist. We did the work-up and we did the blood chemistries, imaging, and everything. There didn't seem to be any warning signs. He saw his family doctor and his family doctor told him the same thing. That patient came back a year later, "I know I have cancer! Do the work-up!" We did an extensive work-up for years in a row, and eventually the patient came in and said, "I know I have cancer. And they found that I have cancer!" And he said, "See, I told you I have cancer!" It was weird. I thought, "Man, that turned into a self-fulfilling prophecy!" A good thought diet is just as important as a good food diet. They're really, really critical! And you want to surround yourself and do things that are going to help your mental health just as much as your physical health. What you're putting into your system food wise is just as important as what you're putting into your emotions and mental capacity.

WHEN YOU KEEP TELLING YOURSELF THAT YOU ARE GOING TO BE SICK, YOU WILL BE SICK.

As a matter of fact, one of the great lessons that I learned was from a patient. I'm going to call this patient Bernice, not her real name. Bernice came into my office, probably six or seven years ago. She was a nurse and was a little bit better established in life than me, but I hate to use the word older. We don't use the O word (old) in the office. We always say matriculated or established.

She had been through breast cancer treatments twice. They found it a third time. Bernice came into the office and she said, "I'm just tired! I can't handle another round of chemotherapy." She had tumors all over in her system. I told her, "My goal is to give you the best quality of life that you can have. I want you to understand that I'm not a cancer specialist, and if this is your choice, I'm going to do everything to support your health." Over the next two years she came in. We were giving her vitamin infusions, balancing her minerals and her vitamin needs, and looking at hormone tests. We did everything we could to balance the patient, and she made a complete recovery. She's doing fantastic! As we got to one of our reevaluation dates, I said, "Bernice, this is really good that you're experiencing this, but I don't know what I did that would do this. I can't take credit for it. Tell me what else you're doing." And she said, "Well, Dr. West, you're not the only doctor that I'm seeing. I'm seeing an energy healer."

She didn't like acupuncture, so she was having acupressure, she was doing massage therapy, and she was coming into my clinic. She said, "You know what the real key is?" (Since then, I have used this on thousands of patients.) "Every night I get a blank sheet of paper, and I just write out all of my stress and worries on a sheet of paper. And then, I tell myself, It's no longer up to me, I'm giving it to God, and I'm going to bed." She said, "I get up in the morning, and I look at that sheet of paper. And I realize that most of my worries and concerns on that sheet of paper I cannot control...I cannot do anything about it! So, I wad up that sheet of paper and I throw it away. I tell my subconscious, 'I'm throwing away things that I can't control!' And this is how I get rid of my stress!"

I have used that so many times with patients, especially when they can't sleep at night. They'll say, "I'm really tired, and I just can't shut off! My mind is sitting there. It's like a little woodpecker, and I just can't shut off because I'm worried about this or I'm worried about that. I'm worried about my kids, and I'm worried about the economy and the state of the world. Am I ever going to get better? And did I move the sprinkler? And did I turn off the oven?" So I tell them "I want you to take a sheet of paper, and I want you to write out your problems." You can't let anybody else see this paper! And this is not a journal! It's not for you to look at when you're frustrated, and particularly, it's not for your spouse to look at."

This is what I do: I take a sheet of paper, and I write an idea in the left corner and in the right corner and in the middle. I kind of doodle... it looks like this spider anagram. I'm just trying to dump. I'm trying to get rid of stuff in my head. My wife, who is much better in every regard than I am, writes down heart-shaped bullets, perfect handwriting, and perfect grammar. You could publish it in *Good Housekeeping*. She will look at my sheet and say, "Wow! That's really disorganized! That really stresses me out!" And I look at her sheet, and I say, "Oh, my gosh! That's so organized! I would be worried about putting everything in the right order and the sentence structure!" Once I decompress by writing everything on the sheet, if I let her look at it, she will say, "I didn't know you were worried about this patient, or quarterly taxes, or payroll, or your patient education system, or the sprinkler that the boys ran over with the lawnmower!" By saying this, she puts all of my stress back in my mind! So I tell her, "I'm not trying to hold any secrets from you, but you can't look at this!" I get up in the morning and sure enough, there are enormous things that bog down my nervous system and increase my stress level of things that I can't control. I wad up the paper and I throw away my problems.

That's one of the best patient exercises that I've done. It doesn't solve all problems, but it's a really nice exercise to show people that there's no perfect treatment, perfect pill, or perfect procedure to get rid of stress. We can manage stress, but we can't get rid of stress. Stress isn't necessarily a disease; it just makes every disease worse! What Bernice taught me, probably 10 years ago, has been very effectual. Our treatments are, first: get educated, second: handle stress levels, and then third: yes, we have individual treatments and modalities for specific illnesses and disease, however one the main solutions in the clinic is utilizing therapies that work, and therapies that work to build people up, treating the whole body. If you look at the many of current medical treatments, it's an acid blocker, it's an acid stopper, it's a beta-blocker, and it's an ACE inhibitor. These all hide the symptoms and do nothing to cure the underlying problems. We're suppressing and we're mandating function but no one in the healthcare arena, except for a few select specialists, are really trying to build you up and make your physiology optimal. That's one of our main focuses and what makes us unique.

Our motto in the office is "Energy, Balance, and Longevity." If we break that down, one of the biggest reasons I think people get chronically ill is because they run out of energy. They don't have the ability to handle all of their needs: physical, mental, emotional and hormonal. They literally set up a system where they rob Peter to pay Paul. Their body starts borrowing minerals from their tissues. It starts overtaxing their adrenal and their thyroid gland just to run the body processes. Their physiology starts getting imbalanced. Their thyroid is working all the time, so it gets tired and it gives up, and they

OUR MOTTO IN THE OFFICE IS "ENERGY, BALANCE, AND LONGEVITY."

get hypothyroid problems. Their adrenals contribute. They can't manufacture epinephrine and adrenaline. The muscles get tired. Their liver gets overworked. They can't process lactic acid, toxins, poisons and everything that they encounter in our environment. Ultimately that impacts quality of life and longevity.

The solution is first, let's get energy back into the system. The bible in our office is a book called *Curing the Incurable* by Thomas E. Levy, MD, JD. We use lots and lots of vitamin C therapy, because vitamin C is an electron donor. In summary, if we give you lots and lots of vitamin C, we can give you lots of electrons. It's like infusing energy into your system. Everything that we do in the clinic, whether it's the physical medicine, infusions, or oxidative medicine, is to try and get patient's energy to come up. If we get their energy to come up, then that really helps to balance their physiology. We give specific nutrients, protocol supplements, and herbs to balance out any organs that are in distress. When we do that, now we get a better quality of life. When we start talking about quality of life, it is not an absence of symptoms. I think that the Vatican has the best description of the quality of life, "It's the mental, physical, and emotional balance that allows you to do what God put you on the earth to do."

I love that definition of life, because if you're just trying to get rid of symptoms, I'm not the doctor to come to, because I can't compete with over-the-counter medications. Just take a bunch of aspirin every day and all your pain is going to go away. Or take a bunch of prednisone; all of your inflammation is going to go away. The problem with that approach is there's always going to be a piper that has to be paid. Eventually, it's going to catch up with you. Prednisone is a fantastic medicine; it's just not a fantastic medicine long-term. We put those things together: energy, balance, longevity, and use the therapies that work, using the least aggressive, least invasive procedure first. Then, as we need to, we can gradually work up to more extensive procedures. Sometimes people's physiology has changed for so long that the appropriate therapy or intervention is a surgery and medicine. But many times, other health care providers immediately go to that intervention first. That is what's inappropriate and wrong with our medical system.

What is the most important vitamin? The answer is the vitamin that you need! That is the most important vitamin! I do believe that, for the most part, minerals are more important than vitamins because every vitamin has a mineral center. And in some instances, if we have the mineral base, we can make vitamins. But by doing the work-up and identifying what people are deficient in, when you give them the right vitamin, mineral, and the right herbal intervention, a lot of times "miracles happen"!

The reason why I put miracles in quotes is because a miracle by definition is, at least in my world, a fantastic patient outcome. We have some miracles in our clinic, but we have even more expected patient outcomes. When you solve the equation and you give the people the right nutrient, you change the body's function, the symptoms change, and the patient becomes healthy and happy. Many times they'll call that a "miracle," but in the West Clinic that's an expectation.

My dad and I came up with a secret sauce. It's the series of interventions that get good patient outcomes. One of the other problems that we have in healthcare is that we like to follow cookbook medicine. That means if a person comes in, they get an A treatment and/or a B treatment or a C treatment. This happens frequently when we have a really good outcome or expectation. Then the patient will go back to South Dakota or to Texas or to Florida, and their doctor will call up and say, "Hey, what is the protocol that you gave the patient?" I'll tell them, "Well, while they were here, we gave the protocol with the vitamin C infusions, the bodywork and the mind-body healing," but that isn't the protocol that patient stays on forever. The protocol, the special ingredients, is whatever the patient needs to make them better. There's no such thing as cookbook medicine in our clinic. Everybody is different. When you come into the clinic and you're in the IV room or you're in one of the treatment rooms—there is no such thing as a fibromyalgia treatment, there's no such thing as a Lyme treatment. There's no such thing as a Staph infection protocol, or even a neck ache treatment. The protocol is specifically for Michelle or for Jason or for Troy or for Jennifer. Whatever their body needs, that is the protocol. It doesn't seem to be that much of a philosophical difference, especially when it comes to infections. In medicine, we're always trying to kill the bug. We want to kill the bacteria. We want to know which bacteria. Is it Staph? Is it E. coli? Is it a virus? Is it a fungus?

You're always going to come in contact with bacteria, viruses, fungus, etc. If your immune system is working correctly, the immune system neutralizes the bad guy or the foreign invader. And if we make the person healthy, then we can get rid of the chronic infections.

I think it's really important to understand why the patient's coming into the clinic, their expectations, and if they are realistic or are unrealistic. Accountability and expectation are part of the solution. Sometimes people will say, "When I come into the clinic, my expectations are very, very low. If I can get any improvement, I'm very happy!"

I just had an experience happen with a gentleman, about a year ago, where he came in and he was in Stage IV liver cancer. He had exhausted every medical intervention and came to the clinic. He asked, "Is there anything that I can add to my treatment?"

My response was, "I will do everything I can to improve your quality of life, but I don't think it's reasonable to say that we are going to turn this around." He said, "Well, my expectations are that you are going to completely heal and cure me, and then, I'm going to get back to my normal life. I'm going to feel like I felt 10 years ago because I have a desire to live, and I have a positive mental attitude." Of course, on the doctor side, you don't want to squash that, but it wasn't a reasonable patient expectation.

I think he passed away about three months after we started working with him, not because of failure of the treatments we provided. The train had left the station and the physiology was so advanced that it was not possible to turn it around.

Matching patient expectations with your treatments and giving positive affirmations is really important. When we do a reevaluation on the patient and they have improved, you have to make sure that you cement that improvement in with the patient. So many times I think patients want to live up to their doctor's expectations, and when the doctor asks the patient how they're doing, the patient automatically reverts to, "What does the doctor want me to say?" The doctor's response is, "I don't want you to tell me what I want to hear. I want you to tell me how you really are." Then you can make the appropriate changes or interventions.

The accountability factor is to make sure that people understand that, in many instances, health is a choice. If you have a loved one who has a serious medical intervention, and they said, "Well, my loved one didn't choose that." I agree with that, but the patient does have the choice of how that is going to affect them physically and emotionally.

This is tough because sometimes people come into the office and they don't want to get better. They're tired from their healthcare condition or their struggle. It's their inner circle, or their spouse, or their caregiver that wants them to get better. The patient says, "Listen, there are things worse than dying, just let me go." The accountability is really asking, "Are you taking good care of yourself?" I tell people," every time I see you I am going to ask you, how is your diet? Are you taking care of yourself?" We have this funny little ritual in the office, particularly when people realize that they're not fueling their systems correctly. We take them to the checkout counter and I get this old, old clinical nutritional book that my grandfather had in the 1930's. I put it out on the counter and I tell the patients, "I need you to understand something that's really important. Your health is not my responsibility. It's not your mom's or your dad's responsibility. It's your responsibility!" And I have them put their left hand on this nutritional method, and I have them raise their right hand. I tell them, "Promise me that you will take your supplements as we've outlined and that you will eat as best as you can, you will put water and liquids into your system and you will try to get yourself on a schedule because ultimately, it's up to you." The patient is the all-star player. I'm one of the coaches the sideline. We have to make sure that you are running the plays and executing what we are doing on the field so that we can win the game."

8

TAKING CONTROL

THE FIRST THING in helping people take control is knowing the patient's why...what their reason is, and how motivated they are to get better. Some people say they're motivated, but they're not motivated. I've had this discussion thousands of times. They'll call from out of state and say, "Hey, I just want to know what I can do to get better." I start outlining a program and I'll say, "First of all, we've got to make sure that you're putting good fuel in your system. How are you eating?" I have found that our bodies crave schedules. So if we can get you to wake up at the same time every day, I think that's more important than going to bed at the same time. It's also important, and very effective, that you get adequate rest, fuel your system, avoid junk food and don't skip meals. I've had people for whom I've outlined a program say, "Ugh! Well, that's just too much work." My response back to them is, "Well, you're not sick enough then. You're not motivated to change." The patient's why is knowing their expectations and what we are going to do to help them meet their expectations.

Earlier I told the story about the guy that came in with his leg dragging. My expectation was to get him completely better. His expectation was to get off of his dependency of ibuprofen every day. Understanding what makes a patient tick and then knowing what their reasonable expectations are is important because they have to drive their healthcare train. They have to drive that vehicle! And this is kind of hard because of what we call "orders patients." In my world there are only two types of patients. There are either "orders patients" or "options patients". The difference is that some people want to know all of their options. They want you to outline a program to give them education. They're really involved in their healthcare and they make the ultimate decisions. So, I act as an advisor to them. I really like working with those patients because they get really, really good outcomes! These are the orders patients. They're the ones in control! I'm not mandating. I'm saying, "This is the rationale for the treatment. This is what we're going to do." The second type of patient is the "options patient." With the options patients, our conversations go something like this, "Mr. Smith, this is what's wrong. Yes, I can fix it! This is how long it will take. This is how much it's going to cost. This is how we can make it so that it doesn't come back." All patients have those five questions. And then, I ask them, "Okay, how involved do you want to be in your healthcare?" And they say, "I don't know. You're the doctor, just tell me what to do." What you have to understand, from a doctor's perspective, is this: are they "orders patients" or "options patients"? Then what you have to do is tell the patient, "You have to take control of your health. Your health is up to you. I'm an invested party in this process, but you have to decide to drive the train. You have to take accountability for it. And if you make improper decisions, it is up to you to get your train back on the track." I think that's really important. First your expectations and second, selecting the doctor.

Then you have to have some pigheaded discipline and determination to stand up to your inner circle, particularly if it's a treatment where everybody is going the same way. They're all doing this medication. And if you decided that you're going to do something different, you've got to be willing to stand up for that and tell everybody, "This is how I want to be treated." Otherwise, your inner circle can be a significant barrier to your healing. You have to decide what life looks like for you, and I don't know where I get this statement—it's called a "normal life." I think this is really important to understand—how to take control.

The statement goes like this, "You're born. You get no drugs and no vaccinations. During childhood, you have the usual illnesses, but conservative treatment gets you through them without antibiotics or drugs, and you build your natural immune defenses. You don't eat white sugar, white flour, too much meat or cheese, don't drink milk or soft drinks. You concentrate on good foods, fruits, vegetable, and a clean, natural diet, and you never learn to drink coffee or smoke cigarettes. The only pills that you take are whole food vitamins, enzymes, and minerals, which are part of your daily intake, and you drink at least a liter of water every day. In your adulthood, you never get sick. You don't get colds, flus, headaches, diabetes, ADD or thyroid problems, panic attacks, growing pains, or digestive disorders. The only pains you experience are from accidental injury and perhaps you do moderate exercise or a sports activity to maintain mobility and general fitness. Your entire adulthood is spent in a disease-free mode. As you age, your mind gets sharper. You experience no arthritis, cancer, osteoporosis, Parkinson's, or Alzheimer's. And finally, after 80 or 90 years, you flicker like a candle and go out."

The above paragraph shows us that it's important to choose the right doctor. Some doctors say, "That's impossible!" And for them, that's true! So, don't go to them. All of this is possible, and moreover, patients are doing it all the time. So listen only to those that can help you achieve your optimal condition in health, because now you've arrived at this part of the world's development when good health and powerful immune systems are not only advisable, but they are very determinate in your survival. I don't think life is just to survive. Life is to thrive, to live your soul purpose, and to do what God put you on the earth to do. And so, when doctors say, "It's impossible to do this! It's impossible." To me that just says that you have the wrong healthcare provider. I think it's really important for the patient to develop some expectations, and then live up to those expectations. We only live up to those expectations of doctors who are actually living that and giving those services. It's kind of like going to a financial planner. I have financial planners that come to the clinic all the time. They say, "Invest in this."

I DON'T THINK LIFE IS JUST TO SURVIVE. LIFE IS TO THRIVE...

I frequently ask them, "Is this what *you* are doing?" And it's surprising to me how some of these planners are not. I say, "Why would I listen to you?" And a doctor is the same. I think it's really important for your doctor to be healthy! If you go in and you see a doctor who doesn't look healthy, who has subtle skin and a yellow complexion and is telling you that you need to exercise and yet is overweight himself, then how can you expect him to be a steward of your health if he isn't even following the directions that he gives you?

This is really important to my wife and me. I treat chronically ill patients every day, so living a healthy lifestyle, striving to achieve and maintain optimal health is really important to me and my family. Am I perfect in my exercise and diet? No, I do not believe that we can achieve perfection, but we can make the best choices when presented with options.

I ask her, "Why would someone listen to me, if I'm not practicing what I preach?" It goes back to accountability, to understanding the patient's reason, and then explaining what normal health looks like. I don't think there is such a thing as a prescription deficiency disease, where you have to have a prescription to be healthy. I don't think that people need some type of stimulate to be healthy. Having those people either in your life or your inner circle who don't have your same expectations of having your "normal life" is the biggest reason to avoid their influence and their input on your mission.

9

THE HIDDEN SECRETS PLAN

WHILE THERE IS no magic bullet, pill, or treatment for chronic disease there are some cheat codes. The secret to getting someone better is to balance their physiology. Understanding barriers to healing in chapter 5 helps you to understand where to start.

Here's the game plan:

Find out the top priority of the patient. Ask them, "If I had a magic wand and you could go back home without one symptom, what would it be?" Develop a priority list. After the list is complete, look at the whole person and do this:

1. Get to know the patient/doctor. It is my opinion that if you and your doctor don't like each other, then find another doctor. This really impairs healing. Maybe sometimes it's neither person's fault but there's no connection. The doctor that is going to take you to the land of health is the one you connect with. Some doctors tell me that they

don't want to get emotionally invested in their patient. My response is "get out of the healing space." It takes emotional commitment and connection with the patient. When you start treating your patients like your family, then you get to another level of healing capabilities.

One of the best lessons my father, an unbelievable healer, taught me was this: if you are not getting the clinical results you want to achieve with patients, it means you are not loving your patient enough.

I know you can't love your patients back from stage IV cancer, or Lou Gehrig's disease or end stage liver failure, but I have seen a lot of people given up for dead that when you take the all-in doctor approach, miracles do still happen.

2. Respect each other. There is no such thing as a perfect doctor, but guess what? There is no such thing as a perfect patient. If you both try your best, there is a better chance of winning. The respect goes both ways. I respect my patients, their travel through the health care system to get to my office and the research performed to get to the West Clinic. I also expect that they will respect the journey through graduate school, doctoral trainings, and continuing education so that I can best advise them on their condition.

3. Patient history. It has been said that 80% of the diagnosis is from the patient history and yet so many times doctors don't take the TIME to do a thorough history. It so important to know the history of the patient. It helps greatly for the patient to type up their history and bring it to their doctor visit. Here are just some of the important factors:
   a. Was there a trigger to start the patients' symptoms?
   b. When did it start? What makes the symptoms better? Worse?
   c. Triggering factors – trauma, environment, and genetics.

    d. Emotional triggers

    e. What is the medical diagnosis?

    f. Does the patient agree with the medical diagnosis?

    g. What is the medical treatment plan or recommendation moving forward?

    h. What treatments is the patient expecting at this office?

For a full list of the medical history questions, please see our website www.westcliniconline.com and click on the new patient link. Regardless if you are coming here or not, your doctor will appreciate the information and it will help your doctor greatly.

4. Write down a day in the life of you, the patient. I am always shocked when patients tell me that no one has ever asked about their life and what happens on a daily visit. I learned this out of desperation.

Here's what happened. I was asked to give a lecture to a group of small business owners about containing escalating medical costs. The appeal to small business owners is that if they help their employees to be healthy using lifestyle, diet, nutritional supplements, and mind/body therapies like meditation and journaling, they will have less medical expenses. This actually was the genesis of our corporate consulting company called 3Cube.life.

I had a business owner that came up to me afterwards and said, "Dr. West, please help me with my medical costs. I have one employee that is responsible for 80% of our health care costs." I said, "I can help him, send him over." Mistake number one; don't say something you can't deliver. I have tried really hard ever since to not open my mouth and insert foot.

The patient came to the office and I started the patient interview. I asked him why he was here and he said, "I mutilate myself. I think there are worms and snakes coming out of my arms, so I take a knife and dig them out. I have to go to the ER at times to stop the bleeding." That stopped my thought process and everything else I was thinking right in its tracks. "What the heck have I got myself into?" I thought to myself. Then the next thought was, "how do I get myself out of this?" I had promised the business owner I could help, but did he remember that I am not a psychiatrist or mental health counselor? Of course he doesn't know that, because I said I could help his employee! Fortunately, I had practiced with a great physician, my father. I told the patient that I needed to go look something up and proceeded to my dad's office. "Dad, I have got this crazy patient in room #2 who mutilates himself. I told his boss that I could help him, what should I do?" My dad sat there for a minute and then told me exactly what I needed to hear, "Son, you're a doctor aren't you? Go be the best doctor that your patient has ever been to."

I went back to the room. My mind was fluttering and as I was searching my data banks for ways to handle self-mutilation, nothing was coming up. They say that desperation is the best source of inspiration and I am living proof. I decided to go to the fundamentals.

"Gene, (not his real name), walk me through a normal day of your life." It was more or less desperation but I am so grateful for the learning experience that happened afterwards. When I am honest with myself, I think I was just asking him that to get him to talk for a while so that when I told him he was in the wrong office with the wrong doctor, it wouldn't be so harsh as telling him that immediately.

He looked at me and said, "No one has ever asked me that. I have been to 15 different doctors. I have been to four different hospitals. I am taking so many prescriptions that I can't even count them. You must really care about me!" Note to self: patients have been some of my greatest teachers. When you listen and try to understand them, empathize and love them, many times you are the recipient of knowledge and human insight.

This was a typical day for Gene. "I can't sleep because my mind won't shut off but my body is exhausted. I get up at 8 a.m. and head to work. I don't feel like eating in the morning, so I go to work and on the way I get my favorite drink, Dr. Pepper. I take a handful of Rx pills that are in my drawer at work. I don't feel well after I take the pills so I drink more Dr. Pepper. Sometimes I'll snack from the restaurant food where I work and then I go home. I take a whole handful of pills at night and then try to go to bed." If I remember right, Gene was taking 27 Rx from five different doctors.

"The Rx bothers my stomach and the only thing that calms it down is Dr. Pepper. Then I try to go to sleep and I am so tired my body shuts off but my mind hallucinates and I think worms are coming out of my arms so I have to dig them out."

Not knowing where else to go, I said, "How many Dr. Peppers are you drinking?" He said, "A lot!" I said, "How many is a lot?" He replied "Three to four six packs a day."

We got him off the Dr. Pepper and on a normal schedule. As soon as he did that, he needed fewer stimulants. He ended up not needing the pharmaceutical therapy.

I learned through that experience that if you really want to get to know your patient, ask them the following:

- What time do you go to bed? How long does it actually take to go to sleep?
- Do you sleep well, or restless and fitful?

- What time do you arise? How do you feel when you get up in the morning?
- When are you first eating? What is it that you eat? (breakfast)
- When are you eating again? What are you eating? (lunch)
- When are you eating again? What are you eating? (dinner)
- Are you eating before bed?
- What about your liquid intake, what are you drinking?
- What activities would you like to do that are you not doing?
- How do you handle stress and agitating emotions in your life?
- Are you willing to change your daily routine?

5. Balance biochemistry. Evaluate recent blood tests or get current blood tests and use medical nutritional therapy (vitamins/minerals/herbs) to treat blood chemistry deficiencies. For a list of recommended blood tests, see appendix A.

6. Balance biomechanics. Make sure the spine, joints and muscles are at optimal health. It is an essential part of the Hidden Secrets plan to use chiropractic, massage therapy, and physical therapy.

7. Balance energies. This is one of the biggest deficiencies in western medicine. Most doctors think that if you can't feel it, x-ray/MRI it, blood test or microscope it, then it doesn't exist. This is a mistake. Through all cultures there are touch therapists, acupuncture, and reflex work. It may not work on everyone, but what treatment does?

I see great outcomes with acupuncture, acupressure, and magnetic therapy. While it may not help everyone, I do not see adverse reactions to these therapies. In our clinic, we offer these and if they do not provide a positive change, we encourage other modalities until we find one that does.

8. Reset the nervous system. This is enormously important and very

rarely done in the United States. Imagine that your body is a computer and if we called up tech support and said, "Mr. Jones' computer is not working, what should we do?" The answer, "Reboot the system. Turn it off and on again."

Since it's not reasonable to kill a patient and bring them back to life, we found that neural therapy is an amazing healing modality. Addressing and restarting chronic nerve problems is essential for chronic disease recovery.

9. Whole food medical nutritional therapy. Your body needs building blocks and the best source gives the body build blocks – medical nutritional therapy is key. You must be able to ingest and absorb vitamins, minerals, fats and phytonutrients. While each patient is different, there are some common baseline nutrients everyone needs.

10. Take prescriptive medication as needed and in conjunction with a health and functional medicine team.

11. Surgery considerations—when appropriate for the case but as a last resort after all alternative therapies fail.

10

THE BEST TREATMENTS FOR CHRONIC DISEASE

BALANCE, BALANCE, BALANCE on every level. That is the keystone to Hidden Secrets. The outline below is how we treat Lyme, RA, MS, FMS, Lupus, Sjogren's, and everything else on our conditions treated list.

1. Lifestyle therapy first – diet, water, and sleep are first priorities

2. Medical nutritional therapy (vitamins/minerals) based upon blood chemistry

3. Vitamin Infusion therapy. I recommend to everyone that they read *Curing the Incurable* by Thomas Levy MD. We see incredible results with high dose vitamin C therapy

4. Oxidative medicine – this includes oxygen, ozone and/or hydrogen peroxide

5. Neural therapy – this resets the nervous system and retrains the body to be healthy

6. Acupuncture

7. Detox therapies

8. Neural therapy

9. Chiropractic therapy

This is the best chronic illness treatment plan.

Treatment 1	Treatment 2
Review labs Medical microscopy UVLRX therapy IV vitamin injection Vitamin B/C shot Neural therapy Chiropractic	Mind body/healing Nutritional review of nutritional supplementation Hyperbaric ozone IV vitamin infusion Neural therapy
Treatment 3	**Treatment 4**
Daily update on progress Detoxification UVLRX therapy IV vitamin infusion Vitamin B/C shot Neural therapy Chiropractic	Daily update on progress PEMF Therapy (magnet therapy) Hyperbaric ozone IV vitamin infusion Neural therapy

Treatment 5	Treatment 6
Daily update on progress	Acupuncture
Detox	Detox
UVLRX therapy	Hyperbaric ozone
IV vitamin infusion.	Vitamin infusion
Vitamin B/C shot	Neural therapy
Neural therapy	Chiropractic
Chiropractic	

Treatment 7	Treatment 8
Mind body/healing	Acupuncture
PEMF Therapy (magnet therapy)	Detox
	Hyperbaric ozone
IV vitamin infusion	Vitamin infusion
Vitamin B/C shot	Neural therapy
UVLRX therapy	Chiropractic
Neural therapy	

Treatment 9	Treatment 10
Acupuncture	Re-evaluation Day
PEMF Therapy (magnet therapy)	Patient case review
	New blood tests
IV vitamin infusion	Medical microscopy evaluation
Vitamin B/C shot	Nutritional review
UVLRX therapy	Chiropractic
Neural therapy	Long term nutritional plan

This cycle may or may not need to be repeated.

IV Nutrient Therapy

One of the most important treatments for chronic disease is oral, intravenous and injection nutritional medicine. By the time the patients come to our office, they are so depleted of essential nutrients, they cannot heal. It doesn't matter if its fibromyalgia, chronic fatigue, low grade infection or recovery cancer. When people are sick for a long time, they do not have the energy to heal. It takes so much energy to be in pain, have insomnia, stomach problems, chronic sore throat, bronchitis, or severe muscle weakness.

One of the best ways to turn this around is to skip the stomach absorption process and go directly into the vein. This allows us to have great absorption by the cells. This is set up through a concentration gradient which means when there is a higher concentration of nutrients outside the cells, we can drive the vitamins and minerals into the cells.

If you have sick cells, the foods that have vitamins and minerals may not be able to get into the cells or at least with enough quantity to make a difference. By having high concentration of nutrients in the blood stream, there is a much greater possibility of getting the nutrients into the organs and tissues.

Let's say your cells are sick and they can only absorb 10-20% of what they need through your food intake. By skipping the stomach and putting the treatment into your vascular system, we can increase the concentration of vitamins to an enormous amount.

Occasionally a patient will ask me if they can get the nutrients if they take them by mouth instead of IV therapy. The answer is that it may be possible and it certainly takes a lot longer. Usually oral therapy is reserved for maintenance and acute conditions. For chronic conditions, those over 90 days respond so well to IV therapy, I always recommend it.

With chronic disease, you usually need large enough doses that are only effectively delivered through intravenous administration. Cells in your stomach and gastrointestinal system can only transport food and nutrients through your system so fast. Your stomach cannot absorb 25,000mg of vitamin C let alone 100,000mg that is routinely given in IV therapy. Most oral tolerance is around 2,000-5,000mg.

One example of IV versus oral is the diarrhea and stomach distress caused by too much oral vitamin C. This never happens with IV therapy. Thus you can get the benefit of high dose vitamin therapy without the unpleasant side effects of an already sick patient. Another benefit, is that you can only swallow so many pills. IV therapy is the perfect solution in cases where a patient is at maximum pill intake or is not absorbing pills, or just can't swallow them.

The last thing I want to point out for the rationale for IV therapy is that by the time many of the serious symptoms of a chronic disease are apparent, it's too late for oral nutritional therapy alone. This can be complicated by length of your illness, previous medications like antibiotic therapy, antibiotic usage, yeast, bacterial overgrowth and current nutritional deficiencies.

This is my #1 recommendation for curing your chronic disease: IV therapy. Our medical team at the clinic routinely uses the following IV protocols:

1. IV vitamin C at 25-50-75-100-150 gram dosages

2. Chelation therapy

3. Dilute hydrogen peroxide therapy

4. Alpha lipoic acid therapy

5. Myers cocktails

6. Dilute hydrochloric acid therapy

I prefer to do IV therapy twice per week and in a series of 10 treatments. After 10 treatments we perform a re-evaluation to determine if we need to change the treatment plan.

Of note, while most of the time I use IV therapy for chronic conditions, it does have some amazing energy booster and vitality effects for healthy people. I get an IV therapy at least every month because I think it helps me to perform at a very high level.

Intravenous Vitamin C

I am a huge proponent of using high doses of intravenous vitamin C in chronic illness, supportive cancer therapy, chronic infections and immune deficiencies, and also on a semi-routine basis for preventative medicine.

The intravenous treatment of vitamin C has begun to receive headlines in a positive light because of information from the prestigious proceedings of the National Academy of Sciences. In reality, there has always been plenty of information available to both clinicians and patients that sheds light on how high IV doses of vitamin C can fight chronic disease; most conventional physicians are not aware of these or state incorrectly that "vitamin C has already been studied and found ineffective." High doses of vitamin C have a pro-oxidative effect rather than an anti-oxidant. This means that vitamin C helps to generate hydrogen peroxide within tissues. This can be selectively toxic to bacteria and cancer cells because the lack of an enzyme called catalase. This enzyme helps to break down hydrogen peroxide into water and oxygen.

These by-products are harmless but in cells that don't have this enzyme, it causes the production of free radicals. This is thought to stimulate programmed cell death or apoptosis in cancer cells. This is one of the reasons that I like to treat patients that have cancer, patients that are recovering from cancer and those that wish to be pro-active in cancer prevention. There are several studies that point out that vitamin C helps to improve the efficacy of chemotherapy and radiation and does not cancel them out.

While most patients are given 25-100g, on serious illness patients I have collaborated with Dr. Thom Levy, the author of *Curing the Incurable* in giving up to 300g per treatment. While this treatment takes 8 hours, most treatments take 45 minutes to 3 hours depending on the dose of vitamin C given.

Dr. Levy's book that I reference, *Curing the Incurable*, has been one of the most important medical texts I have ever read. While IV vitamin C has not cured everyone's symptoms, I routinely see amazing outcomes.

ONE OF THE BEST THINGS ABOUT IV VITAMIN C IS THAT IN MY EXPERIENCE IT IS TRULY NON-TOXIC.

One of the best things about IV vitamin C is that in my experience it is truly non-toxic. Usually when a therapy has the potential to be a great benefit, if used incorrectly it has the potential to harm a patient. Infrequently, I see some nausea (this can be prevented by eating during and before treatment), thirst, urination and rarely some vein irritation. I do not see adverse reactions to vitamin C therapy.

Oxidative Therapies - Oxygen 0_2, Ozone 0_3, and Hydrogen Peroxide

I am still fighting with some chemists who say that ozone is always toxic and should not be used in medicine. Their opinion is based on a lack of understanding about biology and medicine.

~ Velio Bocci, MD, Professor of Physiology at the University of Siena, Italy

The importance of getting oxygen into the body of those afflicted with chronic disease cannot be overstated. The oxygen helps to create energy, reduce acid build up, repair injuries and kill disease causing micro-organisms.

The oxygen therapies discussed here hold great promise for treating some of the devastating diseases confronting humanity today. Together, they form the cutting edge of new healing paradigms and are safe, effective, natural and inexpensive forms of treatment therapy. They are:

1. Oxygen

2. Ozone therapy

3. Dilute hydrogen peroxide

4. Insufflation therapy

Getting the oxygen to the right organ and tissue is really the goal of all of the modalities I use in our office. I prefer to use an oxygen/ozone mixture. This is nearly 99% oxygen but when you run oxygen through an electric spark a very small amount of ozone is created. Ozone therapy is vital in treating chronic disease. In nearly every case The Scripps Research Institute has documented that ozone is actually produced by white blood cells (macrophages) in the body to help fight disease.

Ozone therapy has many useful medical uses. It can destroy viruses, yeast, bacteria and abnormal cells. It is very therapeutic for inflammatory conditions like, Irritable Bowel Syndrome, Ulcerative colitis, tendonitis, and arthritis.

The combination of ozone and oxygen saturates the body with oxygen. This helps to remove poisons, toxins and down regulates inflammation. If these pathways are not accessible, the toxic build up can lead to brain fog, dullness, fatigue, and lack of stamina. If this lack of oxygen is chronic, the overall body is susceptible to germs, and makes us vulnerable to disease.

When blood is exposed to ozone it undergoes a transitory oxidative stress necessary to activate biological functions like cellular repair, immune system activation, hormone activation, and cell synthesis. One of the ozone pioneers, Velio Bocci MD, said, "Ozone can mobilize stem cells already inside the body, which can promote regeneration of the body damaged by free radicals."

Oxidative medicine, like ozone and hydrogen peroxide, provide clinical outcomes that are unthinkable with a single drug or mainstream medical treatments. When you increase the oxygen levels, many symptoms start to decrease and the disease risk factors also go down.

With proper training, the potential for side effects is greatly mitigated. One German study found that the side effects of over 5,000,000 ozone treatments was 0.0007 per application. I don't believe there is any other medical treatment that is this safe.

Oxidative medicine has been found to do the following:

1. Increase tissue oxygenation. This particularly helps with chronic muscle pain conditions like fibromyalgia and myofasciitis.

2. They help to liberate energy from sugars, break down proteins and carbohydrates.

3. They increase effectiveness of antioxidants, or the ability to get rid of excess free radicals in the body

4. They help the immune system by increasing production of tumor necrosis factor and interferon, which the body uses to fight infections and cancers.

5. They increase the effectiveness of red blood cell which delivers ox-

ygen and nutrients to the tissues and removes waste products to the liver, kidneys and lymphatic system.

6. They help to neutralize petrochemicals (oils, petroleum, perfumes and cleaners).

7. Oxygen, ozone and hydrogen peroxide are anti-neoplastic which means they help to prevent formation of tumors and lesions.

8. They help to increase red blood cell disassociation with oxygen, thereby increasing the delivery of oxygen from the blood to the organs, tissues and cells.

9. Oxygen and ozone help to kill viruses

10. They stimulate the immune system that helps to fight infection caused by bacteria, viruses, yeast, and fungus.

Insufflation Therapy

One of the best ways to help sick people is insufflation therapy. This is an incredibly cool therapy that acts to oxygenate the entire body through the use of a very absorbable organ, the colon.

Yes, it's a little socially awkward to talk about but we use a very small catheter to deliver ozone to the colon. The catheter is hooked to a bag and then inserted up the rectum. The volume is approximately 250-750cc. Surprisingly enough it does not cause abdominal discomfort or cramping. The ozone bag is gently squeezed and the ozone/oxygen combination is delivered into the colon. In Europe, doctors consider the colon as the third lung because it has the ability to absorb up to 70 percent of the oxygen introduced to it during surgery.

This therapy is the least invasive of all ozone delivery systems. Many doctors remove blood from the patient, ozonate it and then put back into the patient. This therapy is called major autohemotherapy.

A German doctor by the name of Renate Viebhan, who is an ozone authority stated, "Rectal Insufflation is 95-96% as effective as Major Autohemotherapy".

Managing Chronic Muscle and Joint Pain

The answer is not pain killers or over-the-counter medicines like Ibuprofen, aspirin, Tylenol or Aleve. It is prolozone therapy and neural therapy. Let's start first with Prolozone therapy.

Prolozone Therapy is a form of non-surgical ligament and joint reconstruction pioneered by Frank Shallenberger, MD. It is a permanent treatment for many kinds of chronic pain. Prolozone Therapy is derived from the Latin word "prolix" which means to proliferate, regenerate, and rebuild. Prolozone Therapy is so named because the treatment uses ozone to cause the proliferation, regeneration, and rebuilding of new ligament and cartilage tissue in areas where they have become weak.

Imagine you are driving down the road in your car and you hit a pothole. It jars your alignment and makes some of the lug nuts loose. If you are driving around town, you may not notice but if you are driving freeway speeds, the tire will start to rub. Some doctors turn the radio up real loud so you cannot hear the rubbing. This is like giving a pain killer. The only real answer is that you need to pull your car over and tighten up the lug nuts. That is what Prolozone therapy accomplishes. It literally tightens the rubber bands or ligaments.

When the ligaments are too loose the bone alignment is unstable. The bones rub on each other instead of staying in place. There is a sensitive structure around each bone called the periosteum and when the periosteum touch each other, pain and inflammation occur. If you tighten up the ligaments and thereby help to align the joint, then many of the symptoms of joint pain disappear.

There are nerve endings within the ligaments that are also treated with ozone therapy that helps to diminish ligament pain.

Prolozone works by increasing the blood supply and flow of healing nutrients. It also stimulates two types of cells: fibroblasts, which make fibrous, or connective tissue and chondroblasts that make up cartilage. These two types of cells are used by the body to repair damaged ligaments and joints. This increase of oxygen helps cellular repair activity and removes the causes of pain.

The therapy is performed by injecting a vitamin solution into the joint, into and around the ligaments and sometimes into the soft tissue around the problem area. I have seen a night and day difference in one treatment, but most of the time it takes 4-5 treatments every 2-3 weeks. This usually results in the complete absence of pain and symptoms and works even in severe cases like bone on bone arthritis.

Chronic disease symptoms such as tendonitis, arthritis, rotator cuff, carpal tunnel, hip pain, knee pain, herniated discs, chronic headaches, fibromyalgia, TMJ, sciatica, and neuromas respond well to Prolozone therapy. Even previous surgical areas that have been operated on are worth trying because of the nerve, ligament and scar tissue effects of ozone therapy.

Neural Therapy

Let's pretend you have chronic headaches and it has not responded well to some of the conventional therapies like Rx, chiropractic, Tylenol, stretching, massage therapy or plain old aspirin.

If your body was a computer and we called tech support, they would likely advise us to turn the computer off and on, and reboot the system.

Now it's not reasonable to "kill a person and bring them back to life" but there is a way to reboot the nerves and this is called neural therapy.

It was originally developed in Germany by the Huenke brothers. It involves the injection of Procaine, a glycolyzed ester of para-amino-benzoic acid. This helps to hyperpolarize (open), depolarize (close) and repolarize the nerve (re-set). It is marvelous for chronic diseases and particular in the case of nerve memory.

Nerve memory is a term I use in the clinic that describes what happens when a nerve gets injured. I see this with rodeo cowboys. Every once in a while, they will be roping and will get the rope caught around their finger and then the cow jumps up, takes off, and pulls their finger off. The cowboys will come in and say, "My finger is killing me" even though it is not attached to the body. This is called phantom limb syndrome.

Sometimes even when the body part is not attached to the body, the remaining nerve fibers are so traumatized that they continually tell the brain that they are in pain. This can also happen with an organ or tissue that has been diseased for a period of time. It literally forgets how to be healthy. Neural therapy can reset the nervous system and greatly facilitates the return to health.

Neural Therapy is also often very effective for other medical illnesses such as allergies, chronic bowel problems, kidney disease, prostate and female problems, infertility, tinnitus (ringing in the ears), and many other conditions.

Albert Fleckenstein discovered that tissue which has been damaged, especially scar tissue, has a different membrane potential than normal cells. This is like having a battery implanted into your body. Whenever you have abnormal electrical discharge, the cell pumps stop working and you get toxin build up, abnormal sensations and poisons that accumulate in this area. The tissues cannot heal themselves and this is called an interference field. The biggest source of interference fields is scar tissue. Treating the scar tissue with neural therapy has greatly helped many, many chronic nerve problems. Other causes of interference fields are:

1. Infections

2. Emotional trauma.

3. Physical trauma from any type of surgery, accidents, deep cuts, biopsies, childbirth, dental procedures, vaccinations, burns, tattoos, etc.

Resetting interference fields is critical for chronic disease resolution.

Because of the connection of every cell throughout the nervous system, no matter how distant from each other, when the body has lost the ability to regulate itself through abnormal cell memory or interference fields, the body cannot heal itself. When we provide the necessary balance therapy, nutrition, hormone, and nerve reset therapy, the body can heal itself.

The Body–Changing Mind

Psychoneuroimmunology (PNI) is a pretty big mouthful but it's one of the most important therapies that I have ever learned about. I am so glad to be able to offer this therapy in my practice. Even better, it has nothing to do with pain, needles, or IV therapy.

Mind/Body is CRITICAL for achieving and maintaining optimal health. I can say this because I receive the treatment myself every Tuesday morning before I see patients.

It is a way to help the body heal by turning on the healing capabilities of the brain and enhancing the treatments that we are currently performing on the body. It is the only treatment I know that helps the brain heal the body.

I am so fortunate to be able to work with Dr. James Hollingsworth. He is an expert in PNI therapy. He will take you to room 3 and talk to you about your health concerns. Then using body, mind and listening techniques he helps your mind to create an environment where your body responds. This is how it works:

It is a very relaxing and satisfying therapy. You will have a tremendous sense of calm after completing the treatment. The sessions typically last 30 minutes. Then, even more importantly, there is the ability to repeat the treatment through listening to your personalized and customized CD. You will be able to reinforce the treatment throughout the week. When we incorporated this into our practice we have seen some amazing miracles. I think it is very, very important for you.

Yes, there is a cost associated with the treatment but I firmly believe that in the long run you will save a lot of money because this treatment creates integration between the body and mind and ultimately makes it so you will need less visits, treatments, and trips to the clinic.

Chiropractic Therapy

Chiropractic therapy is a health care system that uses biomechanics, biochemistry and the treatment of the nervous system, muscles, joint and organ function. In addition to clinical nutrition, the chiropractic's primary avenue of care is manipulation of the spine and joints.

The spine is an important structure that houses and provides protection for the spinal cord, while providing mobility for the upper body. This dual requirement of strength and flexibility makes the spine a very complex structure, with multiple joints at each spinal segment (the vertebrae) forming the spinal column.

The word chiropractic comes from the Greek words cheir (hand) and praxis (action), and simply means "done by hand." Note that the word chiropractic, while a bit awkward, is the actual name of the profession.

We use chiropractic care for back pain, headaches, joint pain, carpal tunnel syndrome, tendonitis, sprains as well as non-musculoskeletal conditions including allergies, asthma, and digestive disorders. Some chiropractors further specialize in orthopedics, sports injuries, neurology, pediatrics, nutrition, internal disorders, or diagnostic imaging.

A basic philosophy of chiropractic is that *the body naturally seeks the proper balance* among all the systems of the body, and that these systems are meant to work together. A second basic principle is that *proper structure is necessary for proper function*. If a structure is impaired by injury or stress, its function can be adversely affected.

Thus chiropractic focuses on the integrity of the spine and its surrounding tissues as a means to enhance normal human function and health. This is a vital component of treating chronic disease.

Medical Collaboration

One of the most powerful methodologies available to patients is when true medical collaboration occurs. When doctors put their egos aside, and work for the good of the patients, amazing outcomes occur. The secret sauces of *Hidden Secrets to Curing Your Chronic Disease* is taking the medical and alternative medicine treatments and combining them into a master treatment program.

It is our medical team's goal to have patients 1) take the least amount of supplements possible and 2) to have patients take the least amount of prescriptive medication as possible. We are not meant to be walking pill factories, regardless of the ingredients of a pill. If we correct abnormal physiology by balancing every aspect of the patient's life, then the requirements for Rx diminishes if not completely goes away.

One tremendous benefit we can offer those patients that come to our clinic is a true integrative approach, using the best of both worlds. This is how medicine should work. Use the least invasive, least intrusive and least expensive methods first.

11

WHAT CONDITIONS
WE TREAT

MAYBE A BETTER answer for that is to say what we don't treat:

1. Basically anything that needs immediate intervention at the emergency room such as advanced trauma, wounds needing stitches, compound fractures, acute strokes, heart attacks, and traumatic head injuries.

2. Baby deliveries, although we have great outcomes with pre-birth health of mothers, infertility and post-delivery care. We do not deliver babies.

3. Rx pain management

4. End of life hospice

5. Cancer

We excel in the chronic sickness world. My favorite things to treat are:

1. Arthritis (osteoarthritis and rheumatoid arthritis)

2. Lyme Disease

3. Nerve degeneration

4. Stomach problems

5. Female cycle problems like severe PMS and infertility

6. Fibromyalgia

Basically, if you don't have a trauma emergency, deliver a baby, heart attack, or need Rx to live, we treat it. Here is a partial list of the things we treat.

Adult Acne	Dysmenorrhea
Allergies	EBV (Epstein Bar Virus)
Anxiety	Eczema
Arteriosclerosis	Endometriosis
Arthritis	Environmental Disorders
Asthma	Fears
Autoimmune Disorders	Fibromyalgia
Backaches	Frequent Colds and Flu
Bacterial Infections	Hardened Arteries
Candida- Yeast/Fungal Infections	Headaches
Carpal Tunnel Syndrome	Heavy Metal Poisoning
Chronic Fatigue Syndrome	Hypertension
Chronic Pain	Hypoglycemia
Clogged Arteries	Impotence
Constipation	Infertility
Depression	Interstitial Cystitis
Diabetes	Joint Pain
Digestive Disorders	**Lyme disease**

Menstrual Problems

Migraines

Mood Swings

Neck Pain

PMS

Pesticide Sensitivity

Psoriasis

Rheumatoid Arthritis

Sciatica

Sexual Problems

Sinusitis

Skin Conditions

Stress Related Disorders

Thoracic Outlet Syndrome

Viral Infections

Warts

12

IF IT'S SO GOOD,
WHY ISN'T EVERYONE USING IT?

I GET ASKED all the time, if it's so good why isn't everyone using it? My answer is that they should be using it. Too often, people are doing the normal medical treatments because everyone is doing them, not because they are the best outcome. I will get told, "My doctor told me that vitamins don't have an impact on health, what do you think?" My response is, "try not eating for a while and see how you feel."

"My doctor told me that doctors can't really fix arthritis." The only response that seems appropriate is to say, "for your doctor that is true, but I don't live in that world."

I love this description of life and I wish I could give credit to the author of *A Normal Life* but I do not know who wrote it.

- You're born. You get no drugs and no vaccinations. During childhood you have the usual illnesses, but conservative treatment gets you through them without antibiotics or drugs, and you build your natural immune defenses.

- You don't eat white sugar, white flour, too much meat or cheese, or drink milk or soft drinks. You concentrate on whole grains, fruits, vegetables, and a clean, natural diet. You never learn to drink coffee or to smoke cigarettes.

- The only pills you take are powerful whole food vitamins and enzymes and minerals, which are part of your daily intake. You drink at least one liter of water every day.

- Into adulthood, you never get sick: no colds, no flu, no headaches, no diabetes, no ADD, no thyroid problems, no panic attacks, growing pains, fatigue, or digestive disorders, no high blood pressure.

- The only pains you experience come from accidental injury. Perhaps you do moderate exercise or sports activity to maintain mobility and general fitness. You look to the care of your spine.

- Your entire adulthood is spent in this disease-free mode. As you age, your mind gets sharper. You experience no arthritis, cancer, or osteoporosis, no Parkinson's or Alzheimer's. Finally, one day after 90 or 100 years, you flicker like a candle and go out.

The above paragraph may be useful in choosing a doctor.

- Some doctors will say all this is impossible; which for them is true. So don't choose them.

- All this is possible; moreover, thousands and thousands of people are living it.

- So listen only to those who can help you achieve such a condition of living health.

- Because now we've arrived at the threshold of a time when good health and a powerful immune system are not only advisable; they are the very determinants of survival.

MANY TIMES THE REASONS PEOPLE DON'T GET BETTER ARE BECAUSE THEY ARE SEEING THE WRONG DOCTOR.

Many times the reasons people don't get better are because they are seeing the wrong doctor. One of my colleagues, Dr. Shallenberger always asks his patients, "If a traditional medicine has so many side effects, while predominantly treating only symptoms, why does anybody use it?"

Welcome to the business of health care! You cannot patent natural articles like exercise, diet, vitamin C, D3, herbal medicine. I really think if there was a way that pharmaceutical medicine could get a piece of the revenue stream, these therapies would be mainstream. From a business perspective, profit-driven model, you got to hand it to Big Pharma, they know how to run a business.

The business train twists doctors into the business of medicine instead of patient outcome medicine. Again, I know a lot of doctors that are intelligent, earnest, well-meaning and great people but the machine is hard to escape unscathed.

The answer to why people aren't using the treatments in *Hidden Secrets* is because of the profitability. If you follow the money trail, without giving a tithe to the medical world, alternative therapies are not going to be accepted and without acceptance in the medical world, there is no insurance coverage and therefore the machine takes over and pressures the doctor into only providing services that are covered by insurance. In my opinion, it's hard to be a healer when you contract with a third party for the services given to the patient. Every time I have consulted with a doctor that takes his insurance practice into an all cash model like mine, his clinical outcomes go through the roof. When your only responsibility is the patient and you don't have a third party administrator or insurance company, more miracles happen.

My friend Dr. Shallenberger says it like this:

> In order for any treatment to be accepted as mainstream, it has to go through the rigors of FDA testing, and therapies that are not profitable will not be able to generate the bottom line needed for this incredibly expensive process. In this way our system has resulted in a catch 22 situation, whereby the only therapies to be selected for mainstream use will be those that are the most expensive. Ironically, efficacy in this system is not as important as profitability, which is why treatment protocols aimed at symptom improvement rather than disease eradication are especially attractive.

> What could be more profitable than a treatment that eases symptoms while at the same time not curing the problem? This concept is repulsive to physicians and their patients, who would like nothing better than to be able to cure disease, but again I remind you that these decisions are not made by physicians and patients. They are made by corporate boards who respond to stockholders, not physicians and patients.

Therapies like chiropractic, acupuncture, oxidative medicine, and IV vitamin C will remain alternative rather than mainstream and are always going to be fringe to the skeptic because of the FDA/catch 22 of selecting only the most expensive therapies. Still, once you see the miracles of applying lifestyle, biomechanics, biochemistry, and nutritional IV therapy, you will see the miracles happen constantly. The most valuable judge and source of information is the patient and their clinical outcomes. Why I choose a therapy, protocol or treatment is based upon my experience and the experience of my patient base. I always use these criteria in determining a treatment recommendation:

1. Is there a rationale for the treatment? Is there evidence of efficacy? Is there a success story?

2. Would I do the treatment on my family member or myself?

3. Is it safe?

4. Is it cost effective?

The treatments that I recommend to patients meet the criteria. Why are they not used more? They are not profitable to the drug companies.

13

UNDERSTANDING
PATIENTS

A SOLEMN CHARGE to doctor and health care providers is to
teach your patient what you know and share your opinion. My dad
said, "One of the most important things we can do as a doctor is to
provide education and information to the patient, because informed
patients make the best clinical decisions. Patients know what to do
if they have all the information in front of them." Most of the time,
everybody is aware of what is commonly available, like chemotherapy,
surgery, or the routine prescriptive medication, but just because everyone else is doing it, doesn't mean it's the right thing for you. We need
to educate our patients and the people coming to see us on all of their
options. This book is to inform people about their options so they can
make the right clinical decisions appropriate to their condition.

Everybody assumes that you go to the doctor because you're in pain —well, mainly because you're in pain or fatigued. But the real reason why people go in to the doctor is because they've lost something. This is really important when you're discussing the expectations of the patient because people come in and say, "My shoulder hurts!" But that's not really why they came in to the office. They came in to the office because their shoulder hurts and they can't play catch with their grandson, or they can't garden, or they can't golf, or they can't use their computer mouse. They've lost something that's a really important part of their life. That's why they come in to the doctor. I think the worst thing that we can do, on the doctor side, is to continue to ask people about their pain. We're taught to do these visual analog scales, where we ask people on a scale of 1 to 10 where is your pain today? They start off at 9 and then they're at 7, then 6, then they're at 3.

I THINK THE WORST THING THAT WE CAN DO, ON THE DOCTOR SIDE, IS TO CONTINUE TO ASK PEOPLE ABOUT THEIR PAIN.

Every time we ask about their pain, the patient's subconscious is hearing us cement the fact that they're in pain, and it's, "Pain! Pain! Pain!" Instead, our clinic finds out what the patient has lost and we solve that problem—I always find out what the patient is unable to do. Then we concentrate on that every time they come in. I ask, "Well, can you play catch? Can you go fishing? Can you do the activities that you want to do?" What we're reinforcing is good behavior! We are not reinforcing the fact that it's pain, because when the patients come into our clinic, if they just want to get rid of pain, I'm a really expensive alternative to some over-the-counter aspirin or Aleve. We know that if the patient continues taking aspirin or Aleve, it will harm some of their organs. So, we've got to solve the problem, not just mask the problem!

When you have a chronic and unusual disease you're treating and you want to talk to an expert on that disease, just talk to the patient because they've been everywhere! The great equalizing factor that we're seeing more and more, and even in my short 15-year career, is my colleague, Dr. Google! What happens is people get on Google, and it's a double-edged sword. There's some great information out there... there's also poisonous information! But when people come in and they have fibromyalgia or they have chronic fatigue syndrome, Lyme disease, multiple sclerosis, ulcerative colitis, or cardiovascular disease, it's amazing to hear about the things that they actually know and then teach not only me, but their whole doctor treatment team!

One of the problems we have in healthcare is patient accountability. People have to be responsible for their health. I've said numerous times, "It's lonely to have a chronic healthcare condition," which is what 80% of us are eventually going to deal with either as a patient or as a caregiver. Saddle up because someone in your life that you care about is going to face the current health care system.

Once someone gets sick, a lot of confusion usually sets it. You'll receive advice from your medical doctor, your alternative medical provider, your mom/dad, brothers and sisters, cousin, neighbor, health food store clerk, mechanic, attorney and maybe even your CPA. Then there is the good/bad resource of the internet. Sometimes people tell me the craziest ideas they found while researching their condition.

Here is the *Hidden Secret* to curing your chronic disease...hard work and effort by you and your doctor. It takes a lot of effort, investigation, thinking, innovating and the courage to solve complex health care conditions. It's not always easy. You see, one of the biggest barriers to healing is cookbook medicine. You get a diagnosis (name it), then you identify the symptoms (blame it), and then you get the standard Rx therapy (contain it) for life. Well, name, blame it, contain it is not the recipe for getting your health back.

There is no treatment protocol for cancer, Lyme, mononucleosis, MRSA, or multiple sclerosis. However, there is a protocol for Jim, Nancy, or Mary. You have to design the protocol for the individual patient, not the disease.

This is particularly hard in the medical world where everything has to come from a double-blind placebo controlled study. While I am all for research, sometimes there are too many variables in the individual patient care. There's a big difference between a clinician and a researcher. I am a clinician and what I see working in the trenches is that you treat their deficiencies and nearly always improve their physiology. Even with patients that have a terminal diagnosis if you treat what imbalances and causes deficiencies, they have a better quality of life then if you do not.

14

THE MOST IMPORTANT INVESTMENT YOU'LL EVER MAKE

I CAN THINK of no other investment more important than your health. It's a proven career booster, can generate hundreds of thousands of dollars in extra savings over a lifetime and grows more valuable every single year. It is expensive and distracting to have a chronic illness. Nor can anyone put a price on what sickness means to you in terms of pain, incapacity and forfeiture of quality of life.

The investment is called good health. Nothing is more valuable. When you effectively manage your health it produces a return on investment unmatched by any other investment opportunity. It is vital to your happiness. Best of all, you have the opportunity to contribute to this on a daily basis. You are never too poor or too old to donate to this asset. This requires the approval of no one else.

We should all be spending at *least* as much time educating ourselves and dedicating ourselves to healthy lifestyles and diets as we do to any other activity. This saves a tremendous amount of money in the long run.

Think about a time in your life when you were unable to be a producer or contributor to society because you had an acute case of the flu, vertigo or severe migraine headache. You cannot push through with will power. Your health needs constant tending like a well maintained garden. Even if you are not the victim of chronic illness, being the caregiver of a chronically ill person has a costly impact on income and productivity. When you are sick or one close to you is sick, it affects your job, your relationships and your investing strategies. Those that depend on you are also impacted. Family members have to skip work or sacrifice their productivity in order to care for others.

Whether you are the CEO of a Fortune 500 company or the chief executive of your family, the extent to which you do everything reasonable to protect yourself against illness and disability is unquestionably one of the most important financial—yes financial—investments you can make during your lifetime.

There is never a time to let go of your physical and mental fitness. Achieving and maintaining your health will bolster your self-esteem, help you to relieve stress and preserve meaningful and fulfilling relationships. People that are healthy have that healthy glow that is so attractive to others.

Of course, even those of us who take excellent care of ourselves, exercise regularly and control our diets can still become ill. Genetics, environmental factors and accidents are among the most common causes of non-preventable illness.

None of these recommendations in chapter 17, *What I Do to Stay Healthy*, require a Herculean effort or cost a fortune. But each step could set you on a better path to wellness and wealth. Achieving and maintaining optimal health is vital to your happiness.

When it comes to the health care system and insurance, once again, the system is broken. So many people are paying into a system that does not allow them to select the doctor or treatments of their choice. When possible I recommend a catastrophic insurance plan to cover emergencies and pay for preventative medicine. If you have a knowledgeable health insurance agent there are considerations for Health Savings Accounts and depending upon your employer plan, Health Reimbursement Accounts, cafeteria plans, and Flex plans.

While there is coverage of HSA, HRA, and flex plans, my office does not bill nor accept insurance. Our providers and team members work directly for you! If we accepted insurance company claim forms, we would only seem to be working in your best interests, but by law, we would be working for and responsible to your insurance company first, with your best interests a secondary consideration. Insurance companies do not work for you or for us practitioners. They are profit-driven entities that try to control and use you and us for their profit.

We are dedicated to getting the job done for you, not for insurance companies! It's possible you've decided to come to the West Clinic because you've heard that since we opened in 1916 (yes, 100 years ago) that we have been ahead of the curve with science-based natural diagnoses and treatment. If we were limited to diagnoses and treatments approved and covered by insurance companies, we could not be nearly as effective for you, the patient.

WE ARE DEDICATED TO GETTING THE JOB DONE FOR YOU, NOT FOR INSURANCE COMPANIES!

So why doesn't the West Clinic accept whatever is covered by my health care insurance company, and bill me for the rest? The answer has been the enormous amount of paperwork and administrative overhead, which would increase our cost of service to you even further. However, since 2010, there's been a much more practical reason: We don't want to take even the smallest chance of ending up in jail!

This is not an exaggeration. Because of an insurance claim coding dispute with Regence Washington Health, a US physician who used natural-medicine techniques in his clinics and billed insurance was sentenced (October 27, 2000) to 35 months in a federal prison camp and a $400,000 fine, and lost his medical license for 10 years. How could this happen?

In 1996 the Congress of the United States transformed disputes with private health care insurance companies (previously matters for civil litigation in State courts) into potential federal criminal offenses (Kennedy-Kassebaum Law). Yes, that's criminal offenses, with penalties similar to those levied on drug kingpins: asset and property confiscation before trial, fines potentially in the tens of millions, and lengthy jail time. Medicine has become a much riskier profession than is generally recognized!

MEDICINE HAS BECOME A MUCH RISKIER PROFESSION THAN IS GENERALLY RECOGNIZED!

OK, but I've paid for this health care insurance. Can I use it at all? Experience shows that a professional billing service can usually recover much more of your claim than you can. We encourage you to contact a professional insurance billing company—yes, with all the rules and regulations; insurance billing is now a profession! If possible, find a professional health care insurance company billing service knowledgeable about natural health care billing. As professionals, they know in advance how each company is likely to respond, and how to minimize problems.

What will the West Clinic do to help? Keeping in mind that we work for you, not a health care insurance company, we will provide you (or your professional insurance billing agent) up to 15 photocopied pages of your records at no charge. If your health care insurance company wants more than this, we must charge you, not the health care insurance company (in compliance with RCW 70.02.010) a $15 clerical fee, 65 cents per copy up to 30 copies, and 50 cents per copy thereafter. (Please remember, health care insurance companies refuse to pay for their own demands. Using a professional insurance company billing service makes record requests this large much less likely.)

Services never covered by any insurance plan include services such as research projects, Asyra, Vitamin Injection Therapy, Vitamin Infusion Therapy, Chelation Therapy and most types of oxidative medicine. For this reason, we will not provide these records or records of uncovered services to insurance companies. Should you contract with a professional health care insurance billing company, their professionals can tell you promptly which services are more likely to be reimbursed and which will not. However, for a definitive answer, you must contact your health care insurance carrier.

Must I employ a health care insurance billing company? Of course not! You can do the billing yourself, and ask us for the records you need under the terms immediately above. However, we've observed over the years that DIY takes much more time and trouble, and usually results in much less money recovered.

Is the West Clinic connected financially in any way to any professional health care insurance billing company? No! We work for you, not for a health care insurance company or for a professional health care insurance billing company.

In summary: To continue to do the best job possible for you, using the latest in science-based natural medicine, and (since 1916) to minimize our chances of going to jail for doing so, we cannot accept or file health care insurance claim forms. We strongly recommend you work with professionals in health care insurance billing.

15

THE WEST CLINIC HISTORY

ARTHUR ALFRED WEST was a professional musician and was an excellent violinist. His wife, the mother of eight children, was not in good health, so he decided to go to the National College of Chiropractic in Chicago. He left his wife and family in Pocatello and went to school. Arthur Alfred West, a Doctor of Chiropractic, started the West Chiropractic Clinic in 1916 at the beginning of the flu epidemic of World War I. This Spanish Flu claimed the lives of 60 million people world-wide in a year's time.

His oldest son, Henry G. West, went on a Boy Scout camp out on City Creek. He contracted the flu when he got wet during a rain storm. He was bleeding from the lungs and was so sick he didn't care whether he lived or died. A.A. West, DC gave his son two chiropractic adjustments a day and saved his life. As a result of this anecdotal experience Henry G. West went to the National College of Chiropractic in Chicago where his father had gone to school. Dr. Henry had a pre-med certificate from the University of Utah and was planning to go to medical school. Since chiropractic care saved his life he decided to go to Chiropractic College and follow in his father's footsteps. He joined his father in practice in 1930. The office was located on the second floor of Cook Drug Store, now Maar Drug on West Center Street.

In 1941 the younger brother, Arthur D. West, Doctor of Chiropractic, joined the clinic. In 1948 the office moved to 241 South Arthur in Pocatello. Henry G. West, Jr., a unanimous choice all-state quarterback with a full-ride scholarship to Brigham Young University to play football in Provo, Utah was thrown from a horse on a full gallop on to a hard pan road and suffered a back injury and could not walk. From the expert care of his father, Henry Jr. was playing football three days later. After his football career as quarterback at BYU and his degree in pre-med chemistry with a minor in microbiology, Henry G. West Jr., decided to follow the family tradition and went to the Western States Chiropractic College in Portland, Oregon. He joined the practice in 1961. In 1970 the clinic was moved to 1355 East Center in Pocatello.

Jason D. West studied microbiology at Utah State University. He went on to get his first doctorate from Southern California University of Health Sciences in Whittier, California. He is the fourth generation of chiropractic physicians in the West family. Jason never stopped learning and completed another doctorate in naturopathic medicine, a fellowship in acupuncture and a diplomate in nutrition.

16

THE STORY BEHIND MY NAME, JASON

MY DAD HAD three girls and he was convinced that he would never have a boy. He was Henry George West, Junior. When I was born, my grandma was very anxious for me to be named Henry George West, III. Nothing against anybody that's a third, but I'm just really glad that I wasn't named that. My dad said, "One of the biggest reasons was that it was so confusing in our little town to have a Henry George West, Senior (which was my grandfather) "and then, Henry George West, Junior," (which was my dad.) He decided he wanted to name me something related to health. Jason, in Greek, means healer. That's why he gave me that name. I never thought of being anything else; I just wanted to be a healer.

I'm a fourth generation chiropractor and my education didn't stop there. I later finished advanced training in acupuncture, nutrition and a second doctorate as a Naturopathic medical doctor. I absolutely idolized my dad and I wanted to be like him. When my dad would go to the office, I always wanted to go with him. I'd put on a little white coat, I had a pink stethoscope, and I spent a lot of time at the clinic. My dad was very, very motivated to be on the cutting-edge of medicine. He would go lecture for all of these chiropractic schools. Anything within driving distance. I would go with him. He would do these post-graduate programs in Chiropractic Orthopedics and he would drive to Montana, or Salt Lake, or Boise, and I loved going with him.

As a matter of fact, before I even started chiropractic school, I had completed 3 three-and-a-half-year programs in Chiropractic Ortho-pedics. Some of the things I learned didn't stick, but when people would ask, "How do we treat this?" I would remember and think, "Oh, my gosh! I already know how to do this!" I wanted to be just like my father. I never thought of doing anything else. I always knew I was go-ing to go through high school, college, chiropractic school, and I was going to come back and work with him.

I can remember graduating from chiropractic school where I re-ceived the Outstanding Senior Award and the Presidential Award for contributions to the school. At that time I thought, "All right, I'm going to be unleashed on the world!" I came into practice with my dad and he put his arm around me and said, "Hey, Jason, I just want you to know that now is when the real school starts and this is where the rubber meets the road! Every-thing that you learned in textbooks may or may not be true, but when you start working with patients, this is when you really learn what it takes to be a healer!" Of course Dad

"HEY, JASON, I JUST WANT YOU TO KNOW THAT NOW IS WHEN THE REAL SCHOOL STARTS AND THIS IS WHERE THE RUBBER MEETS THE ROAD!"

was right, starting practice was a really big learning curve for me. Everybody thinks, "Oh, Jason, it was really, really easy for you to go in and just take over for your dad." I want to tell everybody it wasn't...it was really tough! My dad was the smartest guy that I've ever met, the best doctor. Of course, I'm a little bit biased. But I would go out and I would work to get people into the clinic. Patients would sit in the waiting room and they would hear the other patients talking about my dad. They would always want to see him! I would get new patients in and they would say,

MY DAD WAS THE SMARTEST GUY THAT I'VE EVER MET, THE BEST DOCTOR.

"Hey, Jason, no offense, but I want to see the real Doctor West." As the third generation Doctor West, He knew how to treat everything! My code word for when people would come into the office and ask me a question that I didn't know, would be, "Hey, I have to go look something up." I would take two steps down the hall and ask, "Hey, dad, the patient's here, and they've got bleeding gums," or "they have high blood pressure. What do I do?" And he would always tell me.

My dad loved to go to court and be an expert witness. He said the reason was because, "I had a captive audience of a judge, a couple of lawyers, and 12 jurors." He said, "They're all going to be in the office as patients because I'm going to educate them on what I'm doing." He was really, really good at it. Everyone wanted him as an expert witness. As he would leave the clinic, he'd say, "I need you to cover me while I'm gone." I'd probably been in practice three months. I can distinctly remember when the first patient came in and said, "I have urticarial vasculitis." I thought, "Man, I don't even know what that is! I'm going to have to go look it up!" The next guy came in and said, "Hey, my teeth were falling out. They were really loose. Your dad fixed them." The next guy came in and said, "I have a really bad congestive liver." And the next person came in...with all of these cases, I had no idea how to treat them!

Finally, at about 2 o'clock in the afternoon, a guy came in and said, "Hey, my back's a little bit crunched up. Can you give me an adjustment?" I remember thinking, "Awesome! I can treat one patient out of all the people that came in!" When dad came back, I said, "Dad, I don't know what school has taught me. I don't know what I'm doing." He said, "Jason, you've heard the story about the master that meets the people down at the beach. He's going to teach them these different things. They walk out into the water, and the master grabs the pupil and puts his head under water and holds him down. When the guy pops up out of the water, he asks, "What did you do? Why did you do that to me?" And the master tells him, "When you want to learn from me as bad as you want to breathe when I was holding you under water, then you're ready!" My dad said, "If you're ready to do that, then this is what you need to do..." He continued, "School only makes it so that you are not a danger to the public. It doesn't teach you how to be a healer."

From that time on I made a commitment: "I'm going to go to a seminar once a month, and I'm going to be relentless in taking additional Continuing Education classes, until I'm as smart as my dad." That was 15 years ago and it hasn't always been something related to healthcare; but I've always gone to either a seminar on book writing, presentations, biochemistry, hormone balance, nonsurgical orthopedics, or acupuncture, just trying to get up to his level. Every Saturday for about three years, we would get done with patients about 1 o'clock. My dad and I would sit and I would ask him questions like, "Well, what do you do for psoriasis," and "What do you do for acne," and "What do you do for...?" Then, I would take notes and put them on 3x5 cards. I would try to memorize what he told me. That was one of the best things I ever did.

We went through about 900 supplements in this same manner, learning about each of them. He would frequently tell people, "Here's vitamin C. Here's vitamin C with boron. Here's vitamin C with selenium." And I would ask, "Why would you give these different vitamin Cs?" He would go into these complex biochemistry pathways, and I would make these notes. I put them all in PowerPoint presentations. The slide would come in and it would say, "What do you do for anemia?" I would write, "These are the procedures that I would do, and these are the supplements that I would provide." That was a really special time, spending countless hours with someone that was a true healer. I learned at the knee of the best doctor ever!

I have a very good career. I have received the Outstanding Senior Award, the Presidential Leadership Award, the Idaho Chiropractor of the Year (twice), I've been in three documentaries, *Doctored*, *Undoctored* and *Breakthroughs*, and have written three books, but I need to tell you about the thing I am most proud of.

I have made the commitment to attend one continuing education event per year. I was memorizing protocols and supplements and everything else my dad had told me about. It was hard work. I can vividly remember one evening after work; my dad came into my office and sat down. He looked at me for a moment and said, "I would go to you now." I said, "Dad, what do you mean?" He said, "You have the right stuff as a doctor. I would let you be my doctor."

The feeling of accomplishment and validation that I received from that comment is one of my most prized possessions and is a dear memory. Dad, I know you have been gone for nearly five years, but thank you for teaching me, mentoring me, and motivating me. Thank you for the family name and the example of an outstanding physician, healer and teacher. I think of you all the time and am so grateful you are my dad.

17

WHAT I DO TO STAY HEALTHY

- **MY RELATIONSHIPS WITH** my wife and children are top priority

- I exercise every day by walking at least 3 miles

- I eat healthy and alive foods, mostly paleo diet

- I drink 80oz of water every day

- I take my supplements regularly

- I do my best to avoid and eliminate negative relationships. With relationships that I cannot avoid, I put strict parameters. If those parameters are avoided, I immediately leave.

- I journal every day

- I read and memorize information important to me.

- I try to play the piano every day.

- I get involved in causes that matter to me and my wife

People ask me what supplements I take. I respond back to them that I don't even feel bad for them if they don't take as many supplements as I do! Here's my program:

1. Vitamin D3, 5,000iu/day. In the winter, I may use 10,000iu

2. Vitamin C, liposomal 4,000mg

3. Whole food multivitamin

4. Chelated mineral complex

5. Essential fatty acids 6000mg

6. Alpha lipoic acid, liposomal

7. Glutathione, liposomal

8. B Complex, liposomal

9. Men's health complex

10. Prostate prevention program

11. Chlorophyll

12. Brain health program

    a. Memory factor RNA

    b. OPC Synergy

    c. GPC Glycerophosphocholine

    d. SAM-e-

13. Immune system activation/support

Preventative medicine treatments:

1. I get mind/body healing every Tuesday morning (Dr. James Hollingsworth, psychoneuroimmunology, PNI).

2. I get adjusted every week

3. I get a vitamin infusion therapy every month

4. I get a chelation treatment every month

5. I work with my biological dentist, Dr. Larry Bybee every year.

18

PROTECTING YOUR DECISION - SECRETARY OF DEFENSE

THIS SECTION IS really important because this is what happens to people when they leave the clinic. One of the reasons they come to the clinic is because someone told them that we help people with complex conditions. We treat them and get positive results when others cannot.

We start the interview process to determine if we are going to select them as a patient and if they are going to select our team as their health care providers. We learn the patient's expectations. And then, after I understand their condition, I give my expectations.

Our team designs a "Secret Sauce" protocol, which meets the needs of the individual patient. It's different for everyone. Our goal is to restore function and harmony, and we want to increase energy levels. We want to balance their biomechanics, their biochemistry and their hormones. We want to have a pathway for their stress and their nervous system decompression. We want them to have healthy relationships and mind/body healing. As we start to walk through that process, it's appealing to so many people. They say, "How come I haven't heard about this before?"

We usually start a treatment program the day they come to the clinic. After they leave, our team has this little joke. Our clinic is right next to a freeway, and no one has questions until they meet Mr. Freeway. It seems like we answer everything and then the patient gets on the freeway and "BOOM!" They have all these questions!

WE USUALLY START A TREATMENT PROGRAM THE DAY THEY COME TO THE CLINIC.

I call this section "this is what's going to happen," because there are stages of truth.

An example about this is the doctor who said, "Ulcers are not due to stress. Ulcers are related to bacteria!" And for 20 years everybody said, "You're crazy! It's stress-related!" Then he did the testing, and 25 years later everybody hails him as a genius because now everybody knows that Helicobacter Pylori causes ulcers. But that wasn't an accepted truth!

It's the same way with one of my medical heroes, Ignaz Semmelweis. He was the first guy who said that washing your hands in between patients is really important to stop the decrease in childbirth rates. All the infections that were killing mothers and babies at delivery were passed between patients from doctors with germs on their hands. And when he suggested it, the doctors couldn't see any germs on their hands. They said that he was totally crazy! He ended up in an insane asylum because he was so medically castigated and persecuted. This is what we need to help you get ready for. Just because you haven't heard of a therapy doesn't make that therapy any less effective! It really just means that you're not educated. When you share what you are doing with others, many times you are going to get told misinformation.

WHEN YOU LOOK AT TREATMENT OPTIONS THAT ARE MAINSTREAM, THEY HAVE TREMENDOUS MARKETING PROGRAMS BEHIND THEM.

When you look at treatment options that are mainstream, they have tremendous marketing programs behind them. Why do you get a statin drug for cholesterol? Because it's on TV all the time and it's in *Reader's Digest*, and it's in one magazine or another that you're reading. If you take control of what is going to happen, you are going to get a lot of grief and questions because it's outside the norm. What I tell patients is, "One of the reasons you get so many questions is because when people don't understand things, they attack them."

And yet, I've found this to happen a lot. The reason they attack your choice in health care is because they're secretly jealous of your courage to do something different. It makes them feel better if you do what everybody else wants to do! It's so important that people have an educated inner circle or support group, or have specific parameters for those groups where they say, "This is my health." I think this is the most important decision people have related to their health. If you don't have your health, you don't have anything!

People often say, "If it was really any good, everybody would be doing it," or "Oh, my gosh! He lives in Pocatello, Idaho! If he was so good, he would not be in Idaho!" My response to that is, "I choose where to live, and the universe comes to me! I have total faith and confidence so if I want to go to Houston, or L.A., or New York, or Washington, D.C., or Chicago, I can have a successful practice! I choose to live in Idaho!"

Another one of my heroes in life is a doctor named Dr. Shallenberger. He practices in Carson City, Nevada, and he's had the most tremendous impact in my life, outside of the influence of my dad. He has had tremendous courage to stand up to the medical system, and anybody that stands up to the medical norm is going to have battle scars, investigations, and unhappy people because it takes courage to stand up for your patient and treatments that work.

What about the safety?

When patients ask about the adverse effects of the therapies we do at the office, it's a little bit of a struggle to tell them that there aren't any. You might get some bruising, but we're putting natural substances in your system. Usually what I tell patients is, "The worst thing that'll happen is that you'll stay the same." That's the worst outcome that I expect from a nutritional therapy. The worst outcome is to stay the same. There must be evidence of adverse effects and there are some interesting discussions on a double-blind placebo controlled study, which is the medical guild standard for a treatment. But one of the things that I tell people is this: "It's hard to do a double-blind placebo controlled study if you're treating individuals, because we're as biologically different as our fingerprints." In order to get people healthy, you have to treat the patient. Again, the most important vitamin for people is the one that they need. It may be vitamin C, B12, B5, or it may be magnesium. It's the one that they're deficient in. All I really care about when I hear a doctor tell me about a therapy or a procedure for a patient is if it helped the patient, anecdotal or otherwise. And I'm so grateful that I was able to learn from a doctor that just cared about the patient outcomes.

It's interesting when you look at diabetes studies. It'll say that, "These diabetes studies are proven to show this percentage of effectiveness when coupled with diet and nutrition." Okay, well, which one did it? Was it the medication or was it the diet and nutrition? Then, they must be cost-effective. The oxidative ozone therapy meets these criteria for any therapy, despite the fact that we've used these therapies literally for hundreds of years in different parts of the world. It is still hardly used in the United States. It's not profitable to the drug company or to medicine, but it's tremendously therapeutic for the patient. When the patient leaves, they've got to have a lot of courage to do something that is not mainstream. They also have to become educated, and the perfect defense against their inner circle or what's going to happen is to get educated on their therapies and remember that they're not making decisions to make other people happy. They're making decisions for them to be healthy!

The ultimate defense to your selection of health care choices, whatever they may be, is your own intuition. If the treatments make sense to you, and you are aware that other people are being helped, then you owe it to yourself to follow your intuition.

It's your health. If people don't like what you are doing, then either tell them it's none of their business or don't even tell them what you are doing. It's not their health, their choice or their commitment. It's easy to be a sideline reporter or a Monday morning quarterback, but it's not their decision. It's yours. This applies to all of your health care choices. Live your life for you, not your friends, parents, spouse or children. I promise that they will have their own opportunities to make health care decisions. That train is coming for all of us.

19

VICTORY – PATIENT SUCCESS STORIES

THIS IS WHAT the end game looks like. This is Vitamin Hope. Vitamin Hope (H) is not a real vitamin. The Vitamin Hope comes from the realization that there is someone here who is going to build you up, who is going to change your function, who is going to treat you individually, and hear some of the outcomes. Whether it's the story of Gay Rolf, Amanda Thompson, Ashley Mcquivey, or any of the other cases that we have, it's big.

It's one thing for a doctor to tell a patient that he can help with their condition. It's another one for the patient to tell the doctor that he has helped their condition. It's really nice to be able to put this section in the book about all the amazing and wonderful outcomes that I've been blessed to be a part of!

When my boys are anxious to go on a motorcycle ride, or a trip, or go do something fun, their mom and I usually say, "Okay, let's get the yard done. Let's get the garage cleaned." When we define what peoples' expectations are, I tell them, "I really want you to reward yourself! This is the victory where you get to your expectations, and then, you need to do something. You need to go on a trip. You need to visit your kids. You need to buy something that you've really wanted. You need to check something off of your bucket list. You need to celebrate your personal victory."

When it comes to achieving optimal health, it's not enough for us to get there. What we need to do is get you to stay there. Patrick Henry said "Freedom is the price of eternal vigilance." Health is the same. You cannot let your guard down. Your lifestyle always catches up with you. Optimal health cruising means that you do some things that are really important.

It's just like a garden. It's just like anything else in life. It takes work to get there. And the reward is being able to be anything that you want to be, perfectly balanced physically, emotionally, and in your relationships.

For your daily dose of Vitamin H, please see our blog www.dailydosevitaminh.com and sign up for our patient victory notification program. You will get the opportunity to see frequent patient success stories.

20

DIET

>=<

THERE ONCE WAS a surgeon general who was asked, "How much of your health is related to your diet?" We know that chronic health-care conditions chew up a majority of health-care dollars in the United States, and they are the major source of chronic disabling sicknesses and diseases. 80% of it is related to diet. This particular surgeon general said, "That is absolutely not accurate! It's 8 out of 10!"

...CHRONIC HEALTHCARE CONDITIONS CHEW UP A MAJORITY OF HEALTHCARE DOLLARS IN THE UNITED STATES...

Anyway, going on to a diet...you are absolutely what you eat. And I always asked people if that's true, "Are you fast, cheap, and easy? What are you putting into your system?" I've heard about all kinds of diets: The South Beach Diet, The Zone, the Oprah diet, the watermelon diet, the cantaloupe diet, the salt diet, the white things diet, the Atkins diet, the modified Atkins diet, the Paleo, the Paleo autoimmune diet, I mean I've heard it all! And I think that there are some important diets that can be specific for people, particularly with ulcerative colitis and Irritable Bowel Syndrome. I love the book called *Breaking the Vicious Cycle*, which shows how to cure these illnesses with your diet. There are some very important dietary characteristics for auto-immune disorders. For people in general, you need to follow the rainbow diet: when you sit down to eat, you should have a rainbow of colors on your plate—some red, some green, some orange. Skittles, Starburst, and M&M's don't count! It has to be plant-based material.

The healthier and more alive the food is that you eat; the healthier

THE HEALTHIER AND MORE ALIVE THE FOOD IS THAT YOU EAT; THE HEALTHIER AND MORE ALIVE YOU WILL BE.

and more alive you will be. We've talked about foods and that you should not eat foods that don't spoil or that have a really long shelf-life because they're full of dangerous chemicals called food preservatives. We need to call a food preservative what it is. A food preservative is an insecticide. It's a chemical that we put inside the food so that little bugs don't eat it. Here's a newsflash to everyone: we're just bigger bugs! So, you want to eat foods that spoil, you just have to eat them before they spoil. The other diet that I tell people about is that they should eat foods that were around a hundred years ago. It's such a good rule to follow, because that eliminates so much of the junk food! There were no McDonald's or Burger King. We didn't have fast foods, pizza, Hot Pockets, or microwave TV dinners a hundred years ago. People say, "Man, that is really tough to follow! It's not convenient for me to not get something quick." I tell them, "Let me give you a different analogy. There's a saying, 'Nothing is for free. There are no free lunches in life.' You are in your car or walking down the road of life, and there is a toll. On the right side, there is a doctor and the medical institutions, and it's really, really expensive!"

When you blow the engine on the one really nice car that you get in life, we have to do a great, big overhaul! And it's really, really expensive to do that. On the left side are the farmer and grocer. You have to pay one of them. It is much cheaper to pay the grocer and to eat right. It just takes effort and time to do that. Or, you're going to pay 10 or 15 or 20 times that on the right side, which is the medical community. You're paying someone! And when it comes to diet, it's not cheap, and it's not easy to fuel yourself correctly, but it is the way to health. In the end-section of the book we have something called "cruise control," or what I call "Patrick Henry health." Patrick Henry's first most famous quote is, "Give me liberty, or give me death!" The second most famous quote is, "The price of liberty is eternal vigilance!" You'll always have to be watching your rights to be free. And the price of health is eternal vigilance. Your lifestyle will catch up with you. There are no shortcuts. You have to exercise consistently. You have to go to bed, and you have to fuel your system correctly, or you cannot be healthy. Those are my general guidelines for diet. I really don't like wheat per se, and I'm getting more and more courageous to tell people it's a huge factor as an inflammatory food. And you've got to be really careful with dairy products.

Then, depending on your individual sensitivities and if you've had multiple chemical sensitivities, you can get very, very specific and do an autoimmune paleo diet or paleo diets. My favorite dietary recommendations are to tell people to eat paleo; eat like a caveman, remembering that those people were wanderers, and they ate meats, fruits and vegetables. They really didn't have time to plant crops and to harvest grains, and when people ask me about grains they say, "Well, the scriptures say that wheat is the staff of life!" I say, I think wheat used to be a really, really good food. And then what happened is we mixed wheat with goat grass, which is a really successful, resilient weed. The farmers love it because their yields went up a ton using that specific type of wheat. The bakers really like it because it makes healthy, very good-looking bread, but it's like putting Super Glue into your system. The only way to health is to follow the best optimal diet for you, which is healthy, alive foods with minimal man-poisoning or man manipulation.

I'm finding out more and more that people are so sensitive to gluten because of what we've done to wheat by mixing it with goat grass. We have these really high gluten levels. Patients will say, "Well, why do I have to eat this way and no one else does?" If we can get them to understand that it doesn't matter who else eats this way. If you can just dial in and accept your responsibility for your health, for you, and not compare yourself to other people, it really makes a big difference in your own internal happiness and in your own health!

21
THE PROBLEM WITH CHEAP VITAMINS

I WANTED TO do a bonus section on supplements, vitamins, and minerals, because this is just like anything else. You get what you pay for. It's so interesting to me when people come in and say, "Hey, I tried that St. John's Wort for depression," or "I tried that calcium from the membership store." I'll ask them, "Where did you get this vitamin?" They'll say, "Gosh, I got 10,000 pills for $0.49, and I can't believe that it doesn't work!" One of my responses is, "It's so important to understand where the vitamin comes from, where the mineral comes from, who's making it because you do get what you pay for!" I see tremendous outcomes with the right vitamin. Again, the most important vitamin is the vitamin that you need, so you need to get a work-up. Most of the vitamins on the market are junk! A perfect example is that we have this thought process of what makes fractures heal and what prevents osteoporosis is calcium. There's this really cheap calcium on the market called calcium carbonate and it is literally too hard for you to use. It's like eating cement! You can get tons and tons of calcium. You can go over to some of the big memberships clubs or stores, or you can go into the nutrition store, or the health food store, and it's really inexpensive, and it's like trying to digest granite! You can't use it!

We have Paul Harvey that gets on the radio, and he'll say, "We should take Citracal because it's twice as absorbable as calcium carbonate." If you get calcium lactate or some of the other types of calcium, what can occur is you can get a lot better absorption from those. You can get much better outcomes, and it's the same when it comes to herbal therapies. The herbal therapies that are really important to be aware of are the components in your supplement bottle. Does it come from the leaf, the stem, the root, or the flower? Often you'll see studies done on Echinacea, or you'll see studies done on mistletoe or milk thistle, and it's the wrong component of the plant! There's no therapeutic value to it. It is really important to get the right thing! It's really, really important to get the mineral that's most absorbable and that's why we've put together a system on our website where we can provide you these different recommendations so that you can get the maximum value of a preventative medicine program.

ALL VITA-MINS...AND ALL HERBS ARE NOT CREATED EQUAL. All vitamins are not created equal, and all herbs are not created equal. If you're buying a vitamin or supplement that is really inexpensive then you are probably not getting the benefits you should. You might ask, "Do you have to have a work-up before you can start taking a vitamin program?"

And the answer is, "No!" One of the benefits that we have, working through the system in our clinic, we've done a century of research and development. If we have something that we're carrying in the inventory, we know that it works. The reason why I can say that with confidence is in the cash-based model, if someone comes into our office asking for a vitamin or a protocol for a condition and we give them a digestive enzyme for their stomach problem, or a mineral for their restless leg syndrome, or a vitamin combination for their brain function and memory and it doesn't work, the patient never comes back. We have had the opportunity to be in the trenches for 100 years knowing what works and what doesn't. I'm really confident in the products that we have on our website and through our office which has stood the test of time. If it hasn't, we wouldn't have it in our clinic!

We call the multivitamin health maintenance program we have our "All-Star Program," our brain function protocol, our restless leg protocol, our immune system activation protocol. We have developed it through 100 years of clinical experience and tens of thousands of patients, and I'm confident you're going to have a good outcome taking our recommended supplements.

22

SLEEPING SANCTUARY

IF YOU CAN'T sleep, you cannot heal.

This is so funny to put in perspective. We think nothing of spending $25,000 to $50,000 for a vehicle that we're in for two hours a day. One of the things I tell people is, "You know what? You spend way more time in your bed than a vehicle! I think you should go spend $40,000 on your bed!" People's jaws drop! I don't even know if there's such a thing as a $40,000 bed, but if you sleep the way you're supposed to, which is seven to eight hours a night, you're going to spend one-third of your life in bed.

So if the average age of the life of a person is 75 years old, you're going to spend 25 years in your bed! Why would you spend so much more money for your car or your motorcycle or your snowmobile, your jet skis, etc. and not spend at least a couple of thousand dollars on your bed? When people actually buy a proper sleeping arrangement, it's so amazing! But it's hard to get people to spend money on something that they're not conditioned to. "Oh, I'd rather have a BMW that I'm going to spend three or four hours a day in, and I should spend $2,000, or $4,000, or $6,000 on a bed?"

That's a little bit off subject, but it's so funny to tell people that their best investment is to get the best bed that money can buy. If you are having sleep problems, this is an important part of your healing process. You may not be able to fall asleep, stay asleep, have restless legs, or feel exhausted when you wake up and it's taking its toll.

Here are some sleeping sanctuary suggestions:

1. Create total darkness in your sleeping area. This may require black-out curtains or bed repositioning, but it is worth it. Think of it like a bear hibernation area. You go there to sleep, not to work.

2. Take all electronics out of your sleeping sanctuary. This includes LED alarm clocks, TVs and night lights.

3. Consider a grounding pad to discharge electrical build up. It's like a lightning rod for your mind. It grounds the impulses. I have seen great outcomes with this. Look at earthing.com for a sleeping pad that you can put on your bed.

4. Keep a journal. Write down what's on your mind before you go to bed and tell yourself you will look at your list in the morning when you wake up. This helps a great deal for people that can't get their mind to shut off.

5. Positive affirmations and autosuggestion. Tell yourself you can get to sleep and stay asleep

6. Put yourself on a schedule. Don't vary your bed time. It helps to go to bed and wake up at the same time. It puts your body into a rhythm.

7. Consider relaxing classical music, sounds of nature or white noise.

8. Avoid sugar and eating before bed. These habits can raise blood sugar and instead of calming you down will inhibit sleep.

9. If you have hypoglycemia (low blood sugar), do consider eating some natural protein before bed so you can have not have blood sugar drop. This can be a precursor for melatonin and tryptophan.

10. Avoid TV 60 minutes before bed and even better get the TV out of your bedroom.

11. Wear pajamas and even socks to bed. Some people just have poor circulation and by being warmer they will sleep better.

12. Meditate and say a prayer before you go to bed. Try to decompress your emotions.

13. Avoid reading mystery, suspense or horror books. This may cause unintentional stimulation to your brain.

14. Avoid jarring wake up devices. Have a calm alarm clock.

15. Minerals and/or melatonin may be a consideration but should be used with knowledgeable doctor supervision.

16. An hour before midnight is worth more than hours after midnight. Go to bed early.

17. Consider turning off all the power to your house by turning off your breaker box. This works very well for me personally.

18. While you may want to consider pajamas and socks, keep your bedroom cool. Sleeping in too hot of environment can cause sleep problems.

19. Avoid sleeping Rx unless absolutely necessary. The side-effects are scary.

20. Avoid stimulants like caffeine even in the early afternoon.

21. Avoid alcohol. It may temporarily relax and make you drowsy but it does not allow you to get into the deep restorative sleep cycles.

22. Exercise in the morning and try getting your physiology to optimal body weight. Being overweight negatively affects sleep by being a risk factor for sleep apnea and snoring.

23. Reduce fluid intake before going to bed.

24. Take a hot bath, shower or sauna before bed.

25. Don't work in bed.

26. Get the smartphone out of there. It's too disruptive. Put it on airplane mode and put it in another part of the house.

27. Balance out all hormones by going to a good functional medical specialist.

23

Breakthrough & Vitamin H

*I was trapped in my own bathroom for hours, because I could
not turn the bathroom door handle and pull open the door
at the same time, my once strong and functioning hands had
stiffened to mere useless paddles.* ~ Gay Rolfe

TAKING OFF A t-shirt, holding a pen, putting on and wearing ski
boots, and my most favorite passion of downhill skiing, became almost impossible. By late 2005, normal daily tasks suddenly became
very painful for me to do and I was only 53 years old.

The gravity of my symptoms hit me the hardest when I could only
take two downhill ski runs in December. I slept the rest of the day in
my car while my family continued to ski. It was then that I knew my
quality of my life had taken a downward turn, but I didn't know why.

The following day, I went to my family physician. He initially explained my symptoms away as "getting older." Yet, when you live in the Northern Rockies, you know people who hike, bike, ski, and so much more, well into their 80's. It was clear to me that age was not a valid excuse.

On the phone the next day my doctor apologized. My test results had co me back. I tested positive for rheumatoid arthritis and my numbers were extremely high. His first Fix was to offer me oral steroids for the pain until I could see a specialist in Utah. My older sister was diagnosed with Lupus at the age of 39 and died when she was 49. I had seen what steroids did to her firsthand and I didn't like the outcome. I would never take steroids. Knowing that I often used natural remedies and homeo-pathic physicians, my doctor encouraged me to not play around with this serious condition. I needed to see a "real doctor." Even amid the seriousness of my condition, I could not get an appointment to see the specialist until April of 2006, five months away. The rest of the day I cried, thinking about the ski season I would now miss after buying all new gear, and how this illness was affecting my day-to-day life.

With five months to wait before I could see a specialist, I started an online search for help. Most of the information that I found pointed to prescription drugs. Yet one comment caught my attention. "Some-times, for unknown reasons, the symptoms went away." What? I concluded there must be something else out there that had helped people, but went unnoticed by the medical community.

During the waiting period, I went to my holistic physician, saw an-other RA specialist, and started my mornings with a workout routine at a gym. I found that if I kept moving, in spite of the pain and fatigue, I could feel a little better. Even so, my symptoms progressed rapidly. One day I was trapped in my own bathroom for hours because I could not turn the bathroom door handle and pull open the door at the same time, my once strong and functioning hands had stiffened to mere use-less paddles. I was afraid to fully close doors in case I could not get out again. By March, discouragement had settled into my heart. I had more blood work, heard the excuse of "age" again, all while my health continued to deteriorate. I decided to keep the doctor appointment at the University of Utah to get another opinion. I received mixed results, yet the physician encouraged me to start on an experimental drug pro-tocol. "We're not 100% sure what you have, but we feel we should go ahead and treat you as if". The doctors said they could probably help me some, but with my counts so high and as fast as the RA came on, I should expect to be in a wheelchair within two years. The treatment that they had suggested would include chemotherapy, which would cost me a small fortune and could cause cancer. It would make me extremely ill along the way and break down my bone mass. This prog-nosis and treatment recommendation didn't sit well with me because my husband's brother Rex was an ENT doctor and was diagnosed with cancer, a lymphoma. The doctors recommended chemotherapy. All of the bad stuff that they said would happen to me had already happened to my brother-in-law. He wanted treatment with vitamin C, which they would not do. As he was dying he said "the chemotherapy killed me." He was only 31 years old.

The prognosis and treatment recommendation didn't sit well with me. I wanted to save my joints. Why would I want to take anything that would cause me to lose bone mass? Why would I want to further compromise my already weakened immune system and increase my chances of cancer?

I walked away and did not fill the prescription, even though my RA factor was off the charts. While at a local gym, a friend encouraged me to go to the West Clinic in Pocatello, Idaho, just an hour from my home. The clinic had recently started using intravenous [IV] therapies and other cutting-edge therapies like Prolozone and PRP injections, both to help their patients with incurable health and chronic joint issues. I figured I didn't have anything to lose by going and my friend even drove me to the clinic.

The late Dr. Henry West, DC., NMD looked over my blood work. My RA factor was 4600, when it should have been under 80. Dr. Henry West was convinced he and his son, Dr. Jason West, DC, NMD could help balance my body chemistry, to allow my body to heal itself and restore my health.

This was the hope I was searching for! Dr. J started me on a weekly IV protocol of 80% chelation and 20% vitamin C. I also received prolotherapy to help strengthen my joints. I also eliminated most of the sugar from my diet and I increased my consumption of fresh greens.

I am not sure when I started to notice my most dramatic results, but by the spring of 2007, I decided to train for the swimming leg of a triathlon with my daughter. I knew running would be too hard on my joints at that time, but I could swim. The lake near my home became my training ground for the August triathlon and instead of being in a wheelchair by 2008, I participated in this same event in 2007, 2008, 2009, 2010, 2011, and 2012! Then in 2012 I severally damaged my arm skiing and was told there was no hope. Of course the clinic healed my arm...but that's another story.

I am thankful for every minute of every day that I am able to do the things I like. There are some painful times, but I do not focus on them.

I, like so many others who choose the natural medicine route for wellness, realized that it would take time to reverse what took years for the body to create. My treatment plan was not a quick or easy fix, and it required dedication to complete the course of treatment. Yet, without a doubt, I feel this option offered me more complete healing, from the inside out. I am not in a wheelchair, and I didn't have to deal with the dangerous side effects of the prescription drugs or chemotherapy. Along with swimming, I golf (disclaimer: not well) ride my bike and walk 5k races and go ATV riding in the mountains.

I cannot thank the West Clinic team and Dr. Jason West enough for what we have been able to accomplish. The wonderful thing now is knowing I can continue to go to the West Clinic and get a recharge of whatever treatment I need anytime I need it.

Dr. Jason West said, "With any disease process, the only way to treat people is to determine what system, organ, tissue, or biochemical pathway is imbalanced, and then use specific treatments or modalities to balance the body's biochemistry. Balanced people don't get symptoms, pain or debilitating fatigue."

That was key to my treatment—we put all of our focus on restoring my balance and harmony. My determination in getting better along with the focus on restoring my body's ability to heal was key to my outcome.

The RA specialist at the University of Utah said, "We won't need to check your RA counts anymore. You will just have RA for the rest of your life." I had my RA factor tested in July of 2011, my new number 22!

I still love to downhill ski and average skiing 30 times a season—with extra energy!

I hope my story gives you hope!

To see Gays' testimonial please go to: www.dailydosevitaminh.com

24

A FINAL NOTE

I FREQUENTLY REFERENCE my father, Dr. Henry West, in this book. I was so fortunate to have him as a father. He would say, "Love what you do and you'll never work a day in your life." Thank you dad, for the advice and example.

I love being a doctor. I love going to work and I love the patients that I get to see every day. If I won the lottery, I would do exactly what I am doing now.

Wherever you are on life's journey, I hope you or one of those you love will benefit from Hidden Secrets to Curing Your Chronic Disease. I am relentless in learning and discovering therapies that improve the lives of patients. What that means is that this book is going to change.

Please keep up with our latest patient outcomes, discoveries, cookbooks and articles.

- Hidden Secrets to Curing Your Chronic Disease website - www.hiddensecretcure.com
- West Clinic website – www.westcliniconline.com
- Patient testimonials – www.daildosevitaminh.com
- Doctor training – www.drjseminars.com

My family came to this part of the world over a century ago. I have strong roots in the British Isles and served a two-year church mission there. I found this poem there:

May the road rise up to meet you.

May the wind be always at your back.

May the sun shine warm upon your face;

The rains fall soft upon your fields and until we meet again,

May God hold you in the palm of His hand.

All the best in you and your loved ones' health journey,

Dr. Jason West

STAYING HEALTHY, I JUST WANT TO STAY HEALTHY

Follow the rules

1. Put your body on a schedule

2. Sleeping sanctuary

3. Good relationships

4. Manage stress

5. Nervous system decompression

6. Exercise

7. Good food

8. Water

9. Nutritional medicine

10. Schedule down time

Rules of health care

The rules of health in the office are: "Good Food! Good Sleep! Good Oxygen!" If we actually can solve those equations and get people to address them, then we can reverse chronic problems.

APPENDIX A – STARTING BLOOD TESTS

These are blood tests recommended to start on your road back to health. Any tests over 6 months old, I would recommend getting a new baseline, or new tests.

1. Complete Blood Cell Count with auto differentiation

2. Complete Metabolic Panel

3. Complete Lipid Panel (12 hour fast)

4. Thyroid panel – TSH, T3, T4

5. Total iron, ferritin level

6. Uric Acid

7. Phosphorous

8. Vitamin D3

This is a starting place. Depending on your condition, more tests may be recommended.

DR. JASON WEST BIO

Dr. Jason West is the owner of the West Clinic that is located in Pocatello, Idaho. Patients come from every U.S. state and every inhabited continent in the world. The West Clinic was started in 1916, so we celebrate 100 years in practice this year! There have been four generations of doctors and six generations of patients. Dr. West provides treatments for patients who are out of hope, out of time and out of medical options. If you need a boost of vitamin hope please visit our blog, www.dailydoseofvitaminh.com where we continually post some of our amazing clinical outcomes and patient stories. We routinely help people with Lyme disease, arthritis, fibromyalgia, rheumatoid arthritis, MS, and in rebuilding people's health after a serious illness (cancer, traumas and surgeries). Dr. West and the West Clinic have been featured in three health care documentaries, *Doctored*, *Undoctored*, and *Medical Breakthroughs*. He has also written a # 1 Amazon Best Seller, *Hidden Secrets to Curing Your Chronic Disease*, the *West Clinic Cookbook* and a book written specifically for health care providers, *100 Practice Tips from 100 Years in Practice* and is currently writing a book for doctors called *The Destination Practice*.

Dr. West has lectured all over the United States and around the world from Canada to Australia. In addition to his practice at the West Clinic, Dr. West also has a coaching and consulting program for doctors. He teaches other doctors the medical procedures, treatments and modalities developed over the 100-year history of the clinic. In addition, he teaches about clinic culture, business practices and values. Doctors who attend our seminars have increased their patient base, improved patient outcomes and have increased their profitability. For more information, please go to: www.drjseminars.com.

Dr. West is married to his sweetheart, Maxine and has five sons. His family loves the outdoors, snowmobiling and motorcycle riding.

"Personally, I enjoy technology, computers and how they help in medicine. I love to study relationships and communication. People think it takes a lot of courage to see an alternative medical provider and sometimes it does. In today's ever-changing healthcare environment, it takes a warrior to fight the status quo, the establishment, misdiagnosed patients and the standards of care. You have to have courage to be that alternative healthcare provider. I am a strong advocate for patient rights and have gone to battle to protect those rights in their healthcare choices."

~ Dr. Jason West

CPSIA information can be obtained
at www.ICGtesting.com
Printed in the USA
FFHW01n2246071018

9 780997 576238